Praise for *The Plant-Based Dietitian's Guide to Fertility*

This book is a much needed addition to the health and wellness space and relevant to so many more aspects of our health than just fertility. It is a blueprint for healthier living, empowering cou ... ased diet and many more healthy habi ... ugh the professional and personal ler ... iched the content in an accessible and ... nded. **Dr Shireen Kassam**, MB BS, FRC ... ased Health Professionals UK

This book is an authoritative source for everything you need to know about fertility and the surprisingly powerful role food choices play, brought to you with Lisa Simon's expertise and gentle guidance. In contrast to all the medical tests, treatments and other less-than-enjoyable things people do in their quest for fertility, a diet change is enjoyable, enriching and often rapidly effective. **Neal D. Barnard**, MD, FACC, President, Physicians Committee for Responsible Medicine; Adjunct Professor, George Washington University School of Medicine & Health Sciences, Washington, DC

I am so happy that Lisa, an experienced and knowledgeable dietitian, has written such a comprehensive and informative book on fertility from a well-informed plant-based perspective. This book embraces the power of plant-based nutrition and lifestyle medicine and will be an excellent resource for those interested in restoring or optimising fertility. I will definitely be recommending this book to aspiring parents. **Dr Yami Cazorla-Lancaster**, DO, MPH, MS, FAAP, DipABLM, NBC-HWC, author of *A Parent's Guide to Intuitive Eating: How to Raise Kids Who Love to Eat Healthy*

This outstanding book offers both women and men an easy to understand guide to optimising their ability to conceive through evidence-based diet and lifestyle practices. Within these pages, Lisa provides powerful support for a plant-based approach to fertility along with a review of how to achieve adequate nutrition, supplementation, recipe suggestions and lifestyle practices that favour success. These practical tools to improve fertility are based on Lisa's extensive training and knowledge of dietetics, specifically in fertility. An absolute must-read for all those on, or planning on, undertaking, a fertility journey. **Dr Anthony Rafferty**, MB ChB, BSc, MEM, PhD, Integrative Health Consultant

Lisa has an incredible skill for making dietary advice accessible. At a time where nutrition information is confusing and often contradictory, this book provides clear evidence-based information, essential for anyone at any stage of their fertility journey. Lisa offers support, hope and encouragement through her work and it will benefit all her readers greatly. **Dr Laura Freeman**, MB ChB, MRCGP, DRCOG, CCFP, DipOBLM/BSLM, Medical Director, Plant-Based Health Online

This book is a fantastic resource for anyone hoping to conceive either naturally or via fertility treatment. Lisa's style of writing means this wonderful book is accessible to all and her approach to highlighting the benefits of plant-based nutrition and positive lifestyle changes for improved fertility is sensitive and compassionate. What I really love is the mix of her personal tips and advice combined with a strong evidence-base. Highly recommended!
'The Plant Powered Doctor', Dr Gemma S. Newman, MB BCh, DRCOG, DFSRH, MRCGP(2008)

A wonderfully comprehensive and inclusive resource for anyone looking to optimise their reproductive health! Infertility can be devastating for those affected, but Lisa's empathy and positivity shine throughout this book; the personal tone is balanced perfectly with clear, practical, evidence-based advice.
Dr Hannah Short, MA (Oxon), MB BChir, MRCGP, DRCOG, DFSRH, GP Specialist in menopause, POI and premenstrual disorders and co-author of *The Complete Guide to POI and Early Menopause*

This wonderful book is essential reading for all those seeking to better understand and optimise their fertility through plant-based nutrition and other lifestyle measures. It is comprehensive, easy to follow, and meticulously researched, providing much-needed education and practical advice that can be implemented immediately, with the reassurance that all recommendations are backed up by medical evidence. What makes this book even more special though is Lisa Simon's warmth and compassion, that shine through and bring hope to those who are struggling with these issues. An invaluable addition to the literature which I highly recommend.
Dr Zahra Kassam, MB BS, MSc, FRCR(UK), FRCP(C), DipABLM, Oncologist and Lifestyle Medicine Physician; Assistant Professor, University of Toronto, Canada; co-founder and Director of Plant-Based Canada

Lisa is a wonderfully compassionate writer and authority on nutrition and lifestyle for fertility. Her book is backed by the latest scientific research with a holistic approach that seeks to empower readers. If you're trying to conceive or are currently on a fertility journey, this book has you covered every step of the way.
Rohini Bajekal, MA (Oxon), MSc, Nutritionist and co-author of *Living PCOS Free*

This a wonderful book that I will certainly be recommending to my patients and to anyone considering a pregnancy or wishing to optimise their future fertility. Written by a highly qualified dietitian with a clear message, the language is simple, empathetic, and easy to understand. I can see readers being able to apply and benefit from much of the important advice that Lisa Simon explains so clearly throughout the book. This book will empower anyone on their fertility journey, allowing them to take their health into their own hands using nutrition and lifestyle whilst knowing to seek medical advice when appropriate.
Dr Nitu Bajekal, MD, FRCOG, DipIBLM, Senior Consultant Obstetrician and Gynaecologist and co-author of *Living PCOS Free*

THE PLANT-BASED DIETITIAN'S GUIDE TO FERTILITY

From pre-conception to birth

Lisa Simon RD

Foreword by Hana Kahleova MD, PhD, MBA

Hammersmith Health Books
London, UK

First published in 2023 by Hammersmith Health Books
– an imprint of Hammersmith Books Limited
4/4A Bloomsbury Square, London WC1A 2RP, UK
www.hammersmithbooks.co.uk

Disclaimer: This book is designed to provide helpful information on the subjects discussed. It is not meant to be used, nor should it be used, to diagnose or treat any medical condition. For diagnosis or treatment of any medical problem, consult your own physician or healthcare provider. The publisher and author are not responsible for any specific health or allergy needs that may require medical supervision and are not liable for any damages or negative consequences from any treatment, action, application or preparation, to any person reading or following the information in this book. References are provided for informational purposes only and do not constitute endorsement of any websites or other sources. Readers should be aware that the websites listed in this book may change. The information and references included are up to date at the time of writing but given that medical evidence progresses, it may not be up to date at the time of reading.

British Library Cataloguing in Publication Data: A CIP record of this book is available from the British Library.

Print ISBN 978-1-78161-223-1
Ebook ISBN 978-1-78161-224-8

Commissioning editor: Georgina Bentliff
Designed and typeset by: Julie Bennett of Bespoke Publishing Ltd
Cover design by: Madeline Meckiffe
Cover images by: © Tatyana Laputskaya/Shutterstock
Index by: Dr Laurence Errington
Production: Deborah Wehner of Moatvale Press Ltd
Printed and bound by: TJ Books, Cornwall, UK

Contents

Contents

Foreword

The continually increasing numbers of people struggling with fertility issues, and the grief, sadness and suffering that ensue, call for bold action and for taking charge of this important area of our life. With well-researched information and practical tips, Lisa empowers you to do just this, gently guiding you step by step.

I have personally witnessed the anguish of some of my close friends, as well as my patients, after doing everything in their power to have a baby, but to no avail. I have seen their sadness and desperation, and the effects on their intimate relationships. Anyone struggling to conceive is willing to try anything that can alleviate this suffering and Lisa shows how simply tweaking diet and lifestyle has the potential to have a hugely positive impact on fertility, for both men and women.

I am certain that anyone who reads this book will feel confident to move forward in their fertility journey, knowing they are giving themselves the best chance to conceive and, importantly, feeling empowered.

Enjoy this exciting journey!

Hana Kahleova, MD, PhD, MBA
Director of Clinical Research
Physicians Committee for Responsible Medicine

About the Author

Lisa Simon BSc(hons), BA(hons), RD is a Registered Dietitian and studied Clinical Nutrition and Dietetics at Cardiff Metropolitan University for four years before graduating with first class Honours in 2014.

She began her career working in Morriston Hospital in Swansea. After a year working with patients with a wide range of clinical conditions, she took up a rotational post at the University Hospital of Wales, where she worked in Neurology, Cardiology and Respiratory Medicine. She then took up a temporary, specialist post in Critical Care in the Royal Gwent Hospital in Newport, before specialising in Gastroenterology in 2016.

Lisa now works full time at an inpatient adolescent mental health unit as part of a multi-disciplinary team as well as working at CQC (Care Quality Commission) registered healthcare service, Plant Based Health Online, running individual and group consultations and delivering educational webinars. Her clinical areas of expertise are gastrointestinal conditions, liver and pancreatic disease, and male and female fertility.

Lisa has written a clinical update on diet and fertility for the British Dietetic Association and is one of the three Editors of Plant-Based Nutrition in Clinical Practice published in 2022. She is passionate about providing an evidence-based, individualised approach with her patients, using all the pillars of Lifestyle Medicine to enable a holistic and detailed assessment and treatment plan.

Introduction

Why am I so passionate about helping women/individuals/couples to conceive?

Helping others to conceive has been a passion of mine for the last four years and is a result of my own subfertility struggles for many years and subsequent fertility treatment in 2017. I would like to share my story with you to help you understand why I wrote this book and why I feel so much empathy for every one of my patients.

After starting menstruating at the age of 14, my periods suddenly stopped three years later. I was taking a contraceptive pill for acne but I had always had a bleed during the week break so when this stopped happening I was not so much concerned as curious. I spoke to my GP and was referred to gynaecology where I had an internal scan and was told in a fairly blasé manner that I might have problems conceiving later down the line, but I was not given any additional information and I didn't chase it up as I was still a teenager and had far more important things to think about than my future reproductive capabilities.

My cycle continued to be absent over the following years, and although I did occasionally have a bleed, the vast majority of months passed by without one. Still, I never considered how it might affect my fertility as the thought of starting a family had not entered my mind.

When I was 27, I miraculously conceived my eldest son, who is now 14, despite still not having periods, and I assumed at that point that I would have no problems conceiving another child. However, although my periods returned for a short time following his birth, they stopped abruptly again after a few months and it did vaguely cross my mind that I might struggle to have a second child.

Just before my 30th birthday, when I was studying to become a dietitian, I suddenly experienced excruciating pain low down in my abdomen which seemed to be concentrated on the left side. It came completely out of the blue and it was absolutely debilitating; I struggled to even stand up straight, let alone walk. It lasted for a few days and then I was able to resume some sort of normal activity. My GP had no idea what it was and put it down to IBS and as I had struggled with this for some time I accepted it. That was until it happened again a few weeks later with just as much severity and I had to miss several days of uni because I was again unable to walk. As it seemed to be so low down I felt it was something gynaecological rather than bowel related and as it was so severe I didn't want to have to wait for months to be seen so I sought private help, where I was told it was likely to be endometriosis. I ended up having a laparoscopy where endometrial tissue was removed and thought that was it but unfortunately it grew back a few years later and I had a repeat procedure.

My husband and I started to try for another baby several years later without success and after two years of trying we decided to go down the IVF (in vitro fertilisation) route, mainly due to our ages – I was 36 at the time and he was 41. We attended a lovely private clinic – we were not eligible for treatment on the NHS as I had conceived my eldest naturally – and we arranged for the first round of treatment to commence a few weeks later, pending the initial routine blood checks. No reason was found for our inability to conceive and we were diagnosed with unexplained infertility although endometriosis may have played a part.

During this time, and anyone who has gone through fertility treatment will attest to this, I searched for any information that would help to optimise our chances of a successful outcome. It amazed me just how much misinformation was out there, and I felt grateful that having a science background meant I was able to separate out the myths from the evidence-base. One line kept jumping out at me though: a plant-based diet can help to optimise fertility. I also read that a plant-based diet will guarantee pregnancy and 'cure' infertility, and while I knew these were vastly inaccurate claims, I was curious to find out more.

Now I have to admit, when I first started reading about plant-based diets, I was skeptical. I am a dietitian, and I had always been taught that dairy was an essential food group for a range of nutrients, including calcium, phosphate and protein. I had also been taught that meat, particularly red meat, was an important source of iron, so surely removing these foods from the diet would result in nutritional deficiencies and associated disease states, including osteoporosis and iron-deficiency anaemia? As I was soon to discover, and you will read all about these myths over the coming pages, these worries were unfounded.

Having read through many studies showing the likely negative effects of animal products on fertility, and the fertility-optimising effects of plant foods, I chose to eliminate meat, fish and eggs from my diet. However, dairy remained as our first round of treatment was successful and I was concerned about removing major sources of calcium and protein from my diet when my baby was developing. At this point, I still had very little knowledge of plant-based sources of these nutrients. It wasn't until my baby was diagnosed with mild cow's milk protein allergy (CMPA) at 6 weeks and I was breastfeeding that I made the final leap and eliminated dairy completely.

To broaden my knowledge of plant-based diets, I enrolled on the first intake of the Winchester University plant-based nutrition course, run by Dr Shireen Kassam of Plant Based Health Professionals. I found this course to be invaluable, and was quickly reassured by the science that plant-based diets are not only healthier for the planet, but also for the individual in terms of reducing the risk of many chronic diseases.

Interestingly, within three months of going fully plant-based, my menstrual cycle returned and I have continued to have a period every 28-30 days for the past four years. Another welcome effect was the cystic acne that had plagued me throughout my 30s disappeared and has not returned, even during periods of stress which had always been a particular trigger. In addition, I have rarely experienced any endometriosis pain over the past four years, and as an added bonus my symptoms of IBS have pretty much disappeared, although, I'm not going to lie, at first they definitely became worse! It's important I make clear that this is a purely anecdotal story and as a health professional it would be negligent of me to base my advice on my own experience. This is not what I am doing as you will see in the following pages – all the information in this book is evidence-based which means it is backed up by science.

My experience, along with the ever-mounting evidence-base, made me feel very strongly that helping women and couples to reduce or eliminate the animal products in their diets could help to optimise their chances of conceiving. Of course, nutrition is only one piece of the puzzle and there are many lifestyle factors which can also negatively affect fertility, all of which will be covered in this book.

I try to touch on all of these things during a consultation but a consultation only involves one or two people at a time. I want everyone who is struggling to conceive to have this information and to know that there are so many things that you can do to help optimise your fertility. Struggling to conceive makes you feel as though you are not in control of your life but you can take it back; the power is in your hands! Even if you are not trying to conceive, this book will help you to really prepare your body and, if you have a male partner, his too, ready for the day you begin to try to conceive. By laying the foundations, you are not only helping to improve your own health but that of your unborn child.

I have written this book after delving into the science for the past four years and seeing just how much can be done to optimise fertility, not just for women but also for the male partner, father, or sperm donor. Successful pregnancy stories from past patients are the outcomes I strive for and I love to keep in touch with my patients to see how their fertility journey progresses. Hearing that a patient has conceived and carried a pregnancy to term really does make my day, and I have included patient testimonials for you to read.

I also want to highlight that when I refer to 'women' and 'men' I wish to be inclusive and am referring to all individuals assigned female and male at birth as some individuals now may identify as different genders.

So, let's get started!

1

Infertility explained

What is infertility?

The World Health Organization (WHO) defines infertility as 'a disease of the male or female reproductive system defined by the failure to achieve a pregnancy after 12 months or more of regular unprotected sexual intercourse'. There are a couple of issues with this definition. First, not everyone who is unable to conceive has a 'disease' of the reproductive system. Yes, there are certain diseases that can impact fertility, including undiagnosed coeliac disease (more on that later), but for many individuals and couples trying to conceive, there may be many underlying causes for their infertility that do not include any disease state. Second, and I will discuss this more later, the definition is not inclusive of all individuals and couples with infertility.

The term 'subfertility' is also used when describing someone's ability to conceive, and often it is used interchangeably with 'infertility'. However, they are different. Subfertility is a delay in conceiving – for example, if someone has been trying to conceive for a few cycles and has not yet been successful. Infertility is when that delay extends to 12 months or more, so this is the term that will be used throughout this book.

If you have been trying to conceive for more than 12 months it would be a good idea to see your GP or doctor. They will be able to do an initial assessment to check for things that may be causing problems and can then advise you what to do next. The assessment is likely to include questions on your medical history and lifestyle, and may also include a physical examination of you and your partner if applicable. You may then be sent for further tests which, for women, would include blood tests to check hormone levels, scans which can pick up any problems with the ovaries, fallopian tubes and womb (uterus), and any additional examinations that may be needed. For men, tests would include a semen analysis and I will explain what is looked for in this test shortly.

For women aged 35 and over, when fertility is known to begin to decline, infertility may be diagnosed after six months of trying for a baby. This does not mean that when you turn 35, your fertility will suddenly fall off a cliff and you will automatically struggle to conceive. Women conceive and have healthy pregnancies throughout their late 30s and into their 40s and even 50s; it is just that we are born with a set number of eggs and as we age our eggs reduce in number and quality, so conceiving later in life may pose more of a challenge. There is also an increased risk of health problems as we age that may impact fertility, along with an increased risk of miscarriage and genetic abnormalities. That all sounds a bit grim but all I am trying to highlight here is that thinking about fertility-preserving options at a younger age is important and also empowering because if you are armed with knowledge you can then decide what to do with that knowledge. If you fall into the 'older parent' category and have been trying to conceive for six months, do go and see your doctor now. Don't wait for another six months.

How rates of infertility are changing

Almost half of women in England and Wales born in 1989 remained childless by their 30th birthday, an increase of 11% compared to their mother's generation, and 28% compared to their grandmother's generation. This in part is explained by a shift towards delaying child bearing until later years, but it also reflects the increasing rates of infertility in both men and women, which affects 8-12% of couples globally. This is a significant number of people. These fertility patterns are set to continue, with women born in 1995 showing lower rates of fertility in their 20s than previous study populations.[1]

Changing rates of IVF

The game changer for those struggling to conceive came in the form of fertility treatments, which include intra-uterine insemination (IUI) and in vitro fertilisation (IVF) treatment. The first 'test tube' baby, Louise Brown, was born in Manchester in 1978 and since that time fertility treatment has come a long way. A report published by the Human Fertilisation and Embryology Authority (HFEA) in 2021[2] showed in 1991 (when they first started recording information), 6,700 IVF cycles were performed. Fast forward to 2019 and that number had increased to 69,000! Not only that, but success rates have vastly improved as well. In 1991, the chances of having a live birth for each embryo transferred were only 6%. In 2019 that percentage had risen to 25%. There are also significant differences in women in same-sex relationships and on their own accessing treatment. In 2009, 489 IVF cycles involved women in same-sex relationships. In 2019 this had increased almost fivefold, to 2,435, along with a significant rise in IUI treatment. Women going through treatment alone accounted for 565 IVF cycles in 2009, but in 2019 this had increased to 1,470.

Reasons for IVF

Although not mentioned in the 2021 report, the previous HFEA report looking at 2014-2016[3] showed that male infertility was the most common reason for couples accessing fertility treatment. This accounted for 37% of couples. Unexplained infertility accounted for 32%, followed by ovulatory disorder (13%), disease related to the tubes (12%) and endometriosis (6%). The fact that male infertility was the most common reason for couples turning to fertility treatment really highlights how important it is to get men involved in the conversation and making positive changes to their diet and lifestyle in order to help their fertility.

Making the conversation inclusive

It is vital to make the conversation inclusive to all, including those wanting to have a child without a partner, people of colour, people living with disabilities or medical conditions who may require fertility services, those from disadvantaged backgrounds and people from the LGBTQIA+ community.

It is important to make clear that the diet and lifestyle guidance in this book is aimed at men and women without structural defects, such as blocked fallopian tubes, scarring from previous injury or infection, obstruction of the reproductive tract, or congenital defects. In these cases, optimising diet and lifestyle will unfortunately not help to optimise fertility, although it will of course have beneficial effects on overall health and the risk of chronic disease. This book's guidance is aimed at men and women with unexplained infertility, male-factor infertility, infertility associated with hormone-driven conditions, including polycystic ovary syndrome (PCOS) and endometriosis (more on these conditions in Chapters 4 and 5), hormonal imbalances leading to thyroid dysfunction and absent or irregular menstrual cycle, and lifestyle factors including obesity, underweight, excessive alcohol consumption, smoking, stress and poor-quality diets.

I have split the diet and lifestyle advice in this book into what are known as the 'six pillars of lifestyle medicine' (developed by the American College of Lifestyle Medicine). This is because I believe infertility and any health condition can only be helped fully by adopting all six pillars rather than just focusing on one thing. Health is a jigsaw; it needs all the pieces, and Figure 1 sets those out for you.

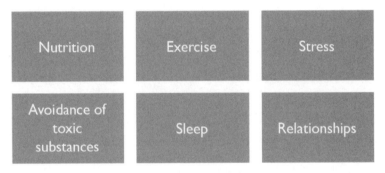

Figure 1: The six pillars of lifestyle medicine

Lifestyle medicine is different from the medical model. The medical model – what your GP and/or gynaecologist will have been taught in medical school – focuses on treating existing diseases with medication but ignores the root causes of many diseases. Lifestyle medicine has six key focus areas: nutrition, exercise, stress, the avoidance of toxic substances, sleep and relationships. It acknowledges that all of these areas need attention in order to treat illness and disease holistically. By highlighting all of the areas in our lifestyle that have the potential to cause ill health, it enables you to take control of your health and encourages positive behaviour change, something that is vital in treating lifestyle-related conditions and diseases. Of course, this does not mean that medication should be ignored; the model is a complementary not an alternative way of treating disease and should always run alongside medical interventions if these are needed. Please run like the wind if you encounter anyone who advises otherwise.

2

The male reproductive system

Male-factor infertility is either a primary or contributing cause in around 50% of couples, but research often focuses on the woman, with the result being we know little about men's reproductive concerns, or how they are involved in their partner's reproductive decisions and health.[1] There are many reasons for male infertility, including injury to the testicles, congenital defects, and inflammation. All of these things can affect the specialist cells in the testicles called Leydig cells which produce testosterone. This is not just important for sex drive but for the whole process of sperm development. Other issues include genetic disorders, the side effects of medications, and problems getting and maintaining an erection. However, I want to highlight that out of that 50% I mentioned, around 40% are not caused by an underlying medical condition but are due to problems with the quality of the sperm.[2] This is important information because it means that in the absence of a disease or medical condition, there may be a solution.

For sperm to do their job of fertilising an egg, they need to be structurally normal and produced in adequate quantities. Although millions of sperm are released during each ejaculation, only one will actually fertilise the egg. When you think about it like that it would be easy to wonder why it can be such a struggle to conceive but, as I will explain, there are many factors involved to ensure that one sperm is healthy enough to make that journey and reach its destination. An individual sperm basically consists of a head, a midpiece and a tail (see Figure 2), and the tail needs to have good movement (motility) to enable it to swim up towards the egg. The overall quality of a sperm determines not just how easily it is able to reach and penetrate the egg, but the health of the foetus that will develop as a result of fertilisation. If all medical explanations for a man's infertility have been ruled out, his inability to conceive may be a result of one or more of the following factors:

- Poor diet quality
- Weight (under or over)
- Stress
- Smoking
- Environmental pollutants
- Alcohol consumption
- Certain prescription medications and recreational drugs.

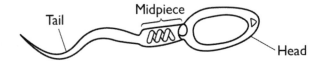

Figure 2: A single sperm

Infertility has the potential to compromise a man's sense of identity, leading to feelings of failure and a loss of masculinity.[3] Including men in the conversation and allowing them to feel as though they can talk about how infertility is affecting them is vital. This may lead to more men seeking help, which in turn can enable them to make positive diet and lifestyle changes to help optimise their fertility. Reproductive health should never be the sole concern of the female because men play an equal role in the conception process. A baby is made half from an egg, and half from a sperm and both need to be of good quality to achieve the best outcomes.

How does the male reproductive system work?

To understand how diet and lifestyle interventions can help to improve male fertility, it is important to first understand how the male reproductive system works.

To start with, it has three functions:

1. To produce, maintain and transport semen.
2. To discharge sperm inside the female reproductive tract to enable fertilisation.
3. To produce and secrete male sex hormones.

Unlike the female reproductive system the majority of which is internal, most of the male reproductive system is outside the body. These parts are the penis, scrotum and testicles, or testes. The scrotum is actually quite clever as it acts as a temperature controller for the testicles. Sperm need the testes to be at a slightly cooler temperature than normal body temperature (about 2ºC less) so to allow this to happen the scrotum contracts the muscles in its wall to move the testicles closer to the body for warmth, or relaxes the muscles to move them further away from the body to allow them to cool. This is why, if the male goes for a cold swim, his testicles will appear to shrink as they move closer to the body for warmth; they are protecting his sperm.

The testicles themselves are responsible for making testosterone, the main male sex hormone, and generating sperm. There are coiled tubes inside the testes called seminiferous tubules and these are responsible for producing the sperm.

There are also internal parts of the system, including the epididymis, which is a tube attached to the testes where the sperm are stored, and the vas deferens, or sperm duct. This is a tube which carries the sperm from the epididymis and towards the penis. When this happens, the sperm collect fluids along the way and this mix of sperm and fluids is called semen. Semen, or seminal fluid, is like a transport vehicle for the sperm, carrying it from the male reproductive tract to the female reproductive tract to enable it to reach its destination.

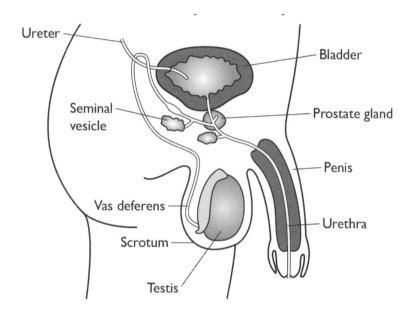

Figure 3: The male reproductive system

You can think of this process in a similar way to planting a seed and watching it grow. In order for the plant to develop, it needs hydration, sunlight and nutrition. Sperm also require these things in order to be of good quality. When I say sunlight, I mean that in a roundabout way. Sunlight on our skin enables us to make vitamin D and, as you will see in the nutrition chapter, Chapter 13, this has an essential role in sperm health.

Male reproductive hormones

Hormones also play a huge part in the reproductive process. The key players in men are testosterone, gonadotrophin-releasing hormone (GnRH), follicle stimulating hormone (FSH) and luteinising hormone (LH).

Testosterone is commonly thought of as a male-only hormone but it is also an important hormone produced in women (I will explain this more in the next chapter). In men it is involved in the creation and growth of the penis and testes, and plays a key role in the development of muscle, the deepening of the voice and hair growth during puberty. It enhances sex drives, is involved in the making of new blood cells, and helps maintain bone and muscle strength throughout puberty and beyond. Testosterone is produced within the testes by the Leydig cells, but also in small quantities by the adrenal glands (small glands that sit above the kidneys). It is essential for the creation of new sperm in the testes, a process called spermatogenesis.

GnRH is released from the hypothalamus in the brain and binds to the back of the pituitary gland, also in the brain. Here it stimulates the creation and release of FSH and LH, both vital for successful reproduction.

FSH and LH work together to produce sperm in the testes. FSH, produced in the pituitary gland in the brain, plays an important part in the function and maturation of another type of cell in the testes, the Sertoli cells. These are essential for sperm production so low FSH levels can really affect sperm quality. LH is responsible for stimulating the Leydig cells to produce testosterone. Low LH levels can result in reduced testosterone levels which not only affects male libido but can also negatively affect fertility. You can see then how important these hormones are for the correct functioning of the male reproductive system (see Figure 4).

Other hormones that can affect male fertility include oestradiol (more on this in the next chapter), prolactin, progesterone and thyroid-stimulating hormone (TSH). I'm not going to delve deeply into these; I just want to mention them so you are aware it is not just the main hormones mentioned above that are present in the male body.

Male Hypothalamic-Pituitary-Gonadal Axis

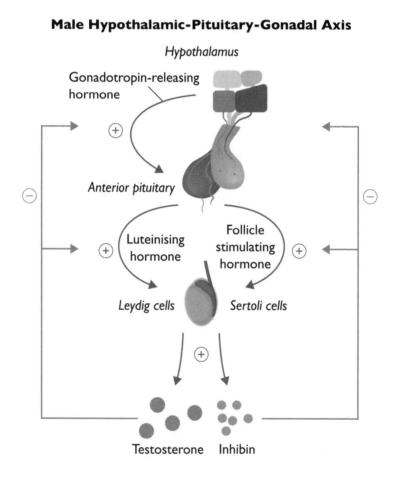

Figure 4: Male reproductive hormones

Sperm quality

There are several different terminologies used when describing sperm quality, most of which have very long names and all sound pretty similar. To save you thinking 'what's that now?!' I've put them in Table 1 so if you come across one of the terms in this book or elsewhere and you can't remember what it means, you can have a quick look here:

Table 1: Definitions of sperm quality

Term	Description
Spermatozoon (plural spermatozoa)	A sperm/sperm
Oligospermia/ oligozoospermia	A low sperm count
Asthenospermia	Poor sperm motility (ability to move)
Oligoasthenospermia	Low sperm concentration and poor motility
Azoospermia	No sperm present
Teratospermia	Low percentage of normal sperm

Men being investigated for infertility alone, or as part of a couple, will need to provide a semen sample and this will then be analysed to check the quality of the sperm. I have set out the healthy parameters in Table 2.

A healthy sperm count is important because, even though it only takes one sperm to fertilise the egg, the more healthy sperm you have, the greater will be your chances of conceiving each month. The volume refers to the amount of ejaculated semen. Motility looks at the movement and swimming power of the sperm: sperm need to travel a pretty long way to reach the woman's fallopian tube to fertilise the egg, so if motility falls below the reference range it can result in male infertility. Vitality looks at how many live sperm are present in an ejaculate, and morphology (structure) refers to the size and shape of the sperm: all men produce some abnormal sperm but the ratio of abnormal to normal is what is important.

Table 2: Healthy sperm parameters as set out by the World Health Organization (WHO, 2010)

Parameters	Reference range
Sperm volume	1.5-6 ml
Sperm concentration	≥15 million spermatozoa per ml
Total sperm count	≥39 million spermatozoa per ejaculate
Motility	≥40% motile spermatozoa or ≥32% with progressive motility
Vitality	The percentage of live spermatozoa must exceed 58%
Morphology	≥4% of spermatozoa

A decline in male fertility

The topic of a worldwide decline in male fertility was first proposed in 1974, and there is a large body of evidence that has been collected since that time suggesting that sperm parameters are declining, especially among young men from general populations in Northern Europe. This includes the UK. A recent study looking at semen analysis of almost 120,000 men between 2002 and 2017 showed that sperm counts declined 10% over that time and the number of men needing fertility treatment increased.[4] Some of the explanations for this include diet quality, weight, chronic diseases such as diabetes and high blood pressure, exposure to environmental toxins, tobacco use, sedentary lifestyles and lack of sleep.[5] All of these factors will be discussed in their dedicated chapters.

Another potential factor that may impact male fertility is the radiofrequency electromagnetic waves (RF-EMW) produced by mobile phones. Use of these devices has increased which has led to much research being conducted regarding their safety. The majority of studies looking at the effects of these waves on sperm quality have been conducted on rats or mice which cannot be used as evidence for the human male population. However, there has been a study on human semen[6] where semen was collected from the male participants and exposed to EMW from a mobile phone in talk mode for 60 minutes at a distance of 2.5 cm from the semen sample. Immediately after exposure, the samples (along with the control samples that had not been exposed) were analysed for sperm concentration, motility and vitality. Although there were no significant differences in sperm concentration or DNA integrity, the motility and viability were significantly lower in the samples exposed to the EMW. There were also significantly higher amounts of chemicals that are linked to chronic inflammation and damage to reproductive cells in the exposed sample. It is important to note that this study had a very small sample size of 32 and more much larger studies are needed. It is also important to note that these will always be test tube studies as, ethically, men cannot be exposed to these waves knowing there might be harmful effects. However, it may be sensible for men to avoid carrying their mobile phones in their pockets or sit with them on their laps.

Inadequate sperm quality is a key contributor to male subfertility, so it is important for the male to do everything he can to produce good quality sperm. This applies to all males involved in the fertility process, from those donating sperm, whether that be for a surrogate or anonymously to a sperm bank, to those in heterosexual relationships.

Erectile dysfunction (ED)

ED is the inability to achieve and maintain an erection, which of course then prevents couples from having sexual intercourse. It most commonly happens after the age of 40 and, as a man ages, the likelihood of ED occurring increases. However, it can also be common in younger men and I have seen patients in mid to late 30s with a number of other health conditions who have been diagnosed with ED.

Is there a cause?

Well, it is commonly a warning sign for cardiovascular disease, with ED occurring about three to five years before a cardiovascular event such as a heart attack or stroke,[7] and, because of this, it is sensible to look at diet and other lifestyle factors that can be addressed to help reduce this risk. These include improving diet quality, reducing stress, ensuring regular exercise, stopping smoking and reducing alcohol consumption. Some medications are also associated with an increased risk of ED, including some antidepressants, antihistamines, blood pressure medications and diuretics (commonly known as 'water tablets'). However, if you are concerned that any medication may be having a negative effect on sexual performance, it is essential that you consult with your doctor as stopping those prescribed for a health condition without medical advice can be very dangerous.

Why blood flow is so important

The penis is an organ of the body and as such relies on a good supply of blood in the same way as other organs, including the heart and lungs. For optimum blood flow, blood vessels need to be in good health so they can dilate (widen) properly and allow blood to flow freely to the penis when a man is aroused. This supply of blood then promotes the contraction and extension of the penis, while the muscles compress the veins, stopping the blood from leaving too quickly which would signal the end of the erection. It's amazing how much blood the penis needs to become erect – up to eight times the amount needed when it is in its flaccid state. So, in basic terms, the aim is to maximise the amount of blood entering the penis and minimise the blood leaving.

The magic of nitrates

One of the most important components of a plant-based diet in improving blood vessel health are nitrates. These provide a source of nitric oxide which plays several roles. It is involved in the relaxation/erection of the smooth muscle tissue in the penis, and also exerts antioxidant, anti-inflammatory effects on the blood vessel walls. Additionally, it helps to widen the blood vessels so that blood can flow more freely to the penis and other organs and this also helps to reduce high blood pressure, which is a risk factor for cardiovascular disease.

So, what foods should men be eating to provide these essential nitrates? Well, leafy greens, berries, pomegranates, oranges and walnuts are among the best sources, but eating a variety of fruit and vegetables will mean a regular intake of nitrates. As our bodies start to lose the ability to make and use nitric oxide as we age, the earlier we start to include these foods in our diet the better. It is worth noting here that sexual dysfunction in women is also increasing, and as a healthy blood supply to the vagina is also important to try and reduce this risk, all of these foods are just as beneficial to women's sexual health. Additionally, a large, recent umbrella review, which is basically a review of reviewed studies (the best you can get), found that including soya regularly in the diet was associated with a reduced risk of vaginal dryness;[8] yet another reason to pack that soya in!

On the opposite side of the scale, animal foods promote oxidative stress in our bodies and this actually reduces how much nitric oxide is available to work its magic. In a nutshell (pardon the pun) this means an increased risk of ED and cardiovascular disease.

Although we don't have published data currently showing that a whole food plant-based (WFPB) diet specifically can help prevent ED, we do have increasing data showing the beneficial effects of a Mediterranean-style diet. Recent research found that a healthful plant-based diet index (hPDI) is associated with a reduced risk of ED, with every unit increase in hPDI being associated with a reduced risk.[9] The hPDI is a way of categorising plant foods that have beneficial effects on your health, so these include whole grains, nuts, fruit, vegetables and legumes, all the foods that make up a WFPB diet. This means that, by including more of these plant-based foods, there may be a lower risk of developing ED. More research is needed in this area but data so far are promising.

So, to summarise: men if you want a happy penis, eat more plants!

3

The female reproductive system

The female reproductive system includes inner and outer parts and these are set out in Figure 5. What I find really surprising is how little as women we know about our outer parts. I carried out a very small experiment and asked a few friends to label both the inner and outer systems on a picture and although all of them labelled the inner system perfectly, not one got every part of the outer system right. This is not uncommon and was found to be the case in a survey by The Eve Appeal, a gynaecological cancer charity in 2016. Less than a third of the women surveyed were able to correctly label several parts of the external reproductive system highlighted in Figure 5, with 44% not being able to identify the vagina and 60% having no idea where the vulva was. This is really concerning, and it also makes me feel very sad. As women, we should know every inch of our bodies, not just to enable us to experience pleasure and to feel empowered, but also to be able to spot any abnormalities that may develop. I would really encourage you to educate yourself on your body (I admit I was one of those women a few years ago) and examine yourself on a regular basis. The best way to do this is by taking a mirror into the bathroom and standing with one foot on the floor and the other on the edge of a closed toilet seat, or something of similar height. Just be careful to maintain your balance and remember to lock the door – the last thing you want is for your partner, or worse your housemate, walking in on you!

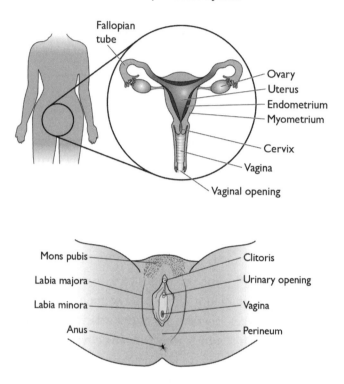

Figure 5: The female reproductive system – internal and external

How does the internal reproductive system work?

A woman's internal reproductive system has several functions including the production of hormones as well as producing eggs and providing the conditions for a baby to develop. It is the ovaries that produce the eggs needed for conception. Each month, one or other ovary will release an egg which is then carried to either the left or right fallopian tube, depending on which ovary produces it. Of course, it is possible for two eggs to be released, which will result in non-identical twins if both are fertilised.

Once the sperm has made its journey to the fallopian tube, its job is to fertilise the egg there. If that happens successfully, the next stage is for the now fertilised egg, the embryo, to travel to the uterus and burrow into the uterus lining. This is called implantation. If fertilisation does not occur, the uterus lining breaks down and results in a woman's monthly period. In order for this whole process to take place, a range of hormones are produced and I will go through these now.

Hormones explained

It can be quite difficult to explain how reproductive hormones work without getting too technical so I hope that Figure 6 will help as a visual aid alongside the text. The key players in women are the well-known oestrogen and progesterone, but also testosterone (though regarded as a 'male' hormone), gonadotrophin releasing hormone (GnRH), follicle-stimulating hormone (FSH), luteinising hormone (LH) and anti-Mullerian hormone (AMH).

As in males, **GnRH** is released from the hypothalamus in the brain and binds to the back of the pituitary gland, stimulating the creation and release of FSH and LH.

FSH: Once this is released from the pituitary gland, it travels to the ovaries in the bloodstream and binds to receptors there, controlling their function. Here it stimulates the growth of the follicles from which eggs are released and increases the production of oestradiol.

Oestradiol: This is the strongest of the three naturally occurring oestrogens and is the main oestrogen in women's bodies. It has many roles but its fertility-specific roles are increasing LH levels around day 12-14 (see below) and thickening the lining of the uterus ready for implantation of a fertilised egg (embryo). It is mainly made by the ovaries and levels are highest when you ovulate and lowest during your period. Oestradiol levels reduce as you age, and this occurs most significantly at menopause.

LH: This travels in the same way as FSH and acts on the ovaries in slightly different ways. In the first two weeks of a woman's menstrual cycle it is needed to enable the ovarian follicles to produce oestradiol. The levels of LH then increase rapidly around day 12-14 to enable the egg to be released in the normal ovulatory process. Once ovulation has occurred, the remains of the ovarian follicle form something called a corpus luteum (basically a structure that secretes hormones). LH stimulates this to release progesterone which is a vital process as progesterone helps to support pregnancy in its early stages. This is why women who go through IVF are given progesterone pessaries following embryo transfer.

Testosterone: In women this is produced in the ovaries and the adrenal glands. It enhances women's sex drive and the majority produced by the ovaries is converted into oestradiol. However, some women can have high circulating levels of testosterone and, although there are several conditions which can cause this, it may be a sign of PCOS and this syndrome will be discussed at length in Chapter 4.

AMH: This is made in the follicles of the ovaries and is used as a measure of ovarian reserve – that is, how many eggs you have. An AMH test when going through fertility treatment will tell you your egg count. A low result suggests a low number of eggs but it doesn't tell you the whole story. It doesn't tell you what quality your eggs are, which is a really important factor, and it has the potential to cause alarm and stress for women and couples going through treatment. As your eggs naturally diminish with age it means that AMH levels will be lower the older you are when you are tested. However, the test can be an important part of fertility treatment as it can be used to predict how many eggs you will produce and what dose of medication to use during the process.

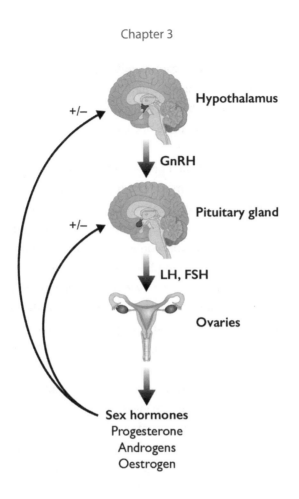

Figure 6: How female sex hormones work together

The menstrual cycle

Just as our pulse is a vital sign of life, the menstrual cycle is a vital sign for reproductive health. A normal cycle is not just the textbook 28 days; it can range from 24 to 35 days, so please don't worry if your cycle is on the lower or higher end of this range. It begins on day one of your period and ends on the day before your next period. There are some situations which may cause temporary fluctuations in your menstrual cycle and these include:

- being on hormonal contraception or other medications
- pregnancy and breastfeeding
- when a woman has recently started her periods, fluctuations in the first year are normal.

Having irregular or absent periods for a prolonged time is a sign that something is not right in your body and I would advise, if this is happening to you, that you speak with your doctor so they can run some tests and refer you to the right specialist to investigate further if needed. It can be especially common in women who do a lot of strength training, to the extent that body fat is stripped right back. Externally these women can appear very fit and healthy but actually with that little body fat comes the very real risk of an absent or very irregular menstrual cycle, and that can cause all sorts of problems, not just for fertility but also for general health. I will discuss this in detail in Chapter 14.

Periods are different from person to person and there can be fluctuations in length and heaviness of the bleed. This happens from time to time and has likely happened to every woman at some point. For example, if you experience high levels of stress there may be an effect on your period that month, or you could have started a medication that is known to affect the menstrual cycle. It is normal to experience small changes, but if those changes continue for several months or are very different to your normal cycle it is important to see your doctor where you can ask about any medications you may be concerned about or be referred on for further investigations. When you are trying to conceive, the absence of your period, or a menstrual cycle which is very irregular, can cause a lot of concern and stress. You can feel concerned there may be something wrong which results in stress, and you can feel more stress because you are trying to work out exactly when you are ovulating and trying to conceive within that window. I have been there and I know the pressures it can put not just on yourself but on your relationship.

It is not a fun way to live so please do make sure if you have any concerns about your menstrual cycle you make an appointment to speak with your doctor.

The phases of the menstrual cycle

When women talk about their menstrual cycle it is often very much focused on their period, but there is so much more to it than that. It is divided into two main phases: the follicular phase followed by the luteal phase. Figure 7 shows the differences in hormone levels in the two phases and will hopefully make it easier to understand.

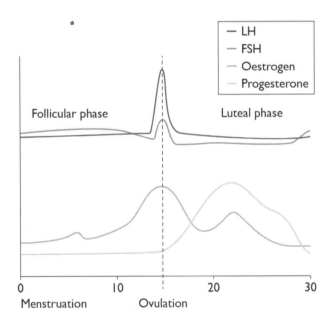

Figure 7: The phases of the menstrual cycle

The follicular phase begins on the first day of your period and ends when you start to ovulate, so it typically takes up the whole of the first part of your menstrual cycle. Oestrogen levels increase and this promotes thickening of the lining of the uterus. FSH levels rise which stimulate the growth of some follicles in the ovary. One of these follicles becomes dominant and produces an egg. You may feel an increase in energy levels, along with greater focus, mental clarity and a more positive mood. I know for me this part of my cycle is when I am the most productive. I can feel the effects on my brain as soon as I enter the next phases – it literally turns to cotton wool!

The luteal phase lasts from day one of ovulation to the day before your period. During the luteal phase, there is a rise in progesterone which works alongside oestrogen to enable the uterine lining to remain thick in preparation for pregnancy. When your body recognises there hasn't been a pregnancy, hormone levels will decrease and this triggers the onset of your period. For a few days during the luteal phase, many women experience symptoms known as premenstrual syndrome, or PMS. These include fatigue, brain fog, lower mood and irritability. During this phase it is really important to be kind to yourself. If you feel like just curling up on the sofa in your PJs with a book and some delicious plant-based chocolate, that's okay! Listen to your body, allow yourself to be anti-social if you don't feel like seeing anyone, and know that in a few days these feelings will pass and you will be back to your old self. If you feel though that your symptoms are taking over and lasting for a significant length of time each month, please seek help as this may be a sign of a menstrual cycle disorder called premenstrual dysphoric disorder, or PMDD. This is similar to PMS but the symptoms, especially the emotional ones can be much more severe and some women can really struggle to function during these weeks, with sometimes huge effects on their home and work life. There are so many things that can be done to make this half of your cycle easier, so please do speak to your doctor and don't suffer in silence.

Primary and secondary amenorrhoea

Amenorrhoea is the term used to describe an absence of your period and there are two types, primary and secondary.

Primary amenorrhoea is when a young woman does not have her first period by the age of 15. Usually, a girl will get her first period around the age of 12, but it can be earlier. I must stress that this condition is rare, with less than 0.1% of the population affected. Causes of primary amenorrhoea include PCOS, premature ovarian insufficiency (POI), anatomical defects and a genetic condition called Turner syndrome which only affects females.

Secondary amenorrhoea is the term used when a woman initially menstruates but then her periods suddenly stop for at least three consecutive cycles if previously menstruating regularly, or six cycles if previously experiencing an irregular cycle. Functional hypothalamic amenorrhoea (FHA) is one of the most common causes of absent periods, particularly in women with PCOS, and can present as both primary or secondary amenorrhoea, but other causes must be ruled out before this is diagnosed. FHA is caused by a functional disorder of the hypothalamus which has an impact on the hormones that it produces. It is potentially reversible and needs to be addressed because if low levels of oestogen continue in the long term, there can be consequences to bone, mental and reproductive health, and an increased risk of cardiovascular disease.

Common triggers for FHA include lifestyle factors that can easily be addressed with the right support. These include excessive exercising, high levels of stress, disordered eating and low body weight. It has often been found to be the underlying cause for absent periods in women who maintain their weight at the higher end of their ideal body weight but who display signs of disordered eating, such as avoiding certain foods or fasting for long periods. This shows that it is not just women who are classed as underweight who are at risk of FHA and the resulting hormonal imbalance; it is any woman who has a disordered relationship with food, and/or is experiencing chronic stress, and/or over-exercising. All of these things can impact the menstrual cycle so if you feel any of these apply to you it is important to mention them to your doctor if you are attending with a history of absent or irregular periods.

Studies have shown that women with FHA may be at higher risk of depression and cope less well with stress, including their autonomic responses. Let me explain.

The effects of stress

The autonomic nervous system consists of the sympathetic (fight or flight) and parasympathetic (rest and digest) systems. When a stressful event happens, the sympathetic nervous system responds by increasing our heart and breathing rates. We become more alert and aware, and our energy levels are increased to prepare us for action. You can feel these effects when you are about to do something you find stressful; you may feel as though your heart has gone into overdrive and you will feel as though you have adrenaline racing through your body. You may also become restless and feel hot. This is your sympathetic nervous system kicking in. In this sense it is a bit of a misnomer – not very sympathetic, right?

The parasympathetic system does the opposite. Once the stressful event is over it brings down our heart and breathing rate, conserves energy expenditure, and the body enters a calm state. You can activate this system yourself by practising meditation, or yoga for example, which is why stress management tools are so important. When both systems work in harmony, the body remains in balance: the sympathetic system gives us the tools we need to respond to stress appropriately and the parasympathetic system returns us back to our previously calm state. The problem occurs when the sympathetic system remains switched on when the body is not coping with stress as it should. This means the body remains in constant fight-or-flight mode which increases the chance of a number of health conditions if it continues for a long time. This includes negative effects on reproductive health.

Cognitive behavioural therapy (CBT) can be useful for anyone who suffers from chronic stress and anxiety, but it has been shown in studies to be effective for women who have FHA related to high levels of stress. CBT is a talking therapy which can help change the way you think and behave as the aim is to reduce negative thoughts and feelings that can leave you trapped in a vicious circle. I bet you will all have experienced this at various points of your life but if it is something that is happening frequently it would be a good idea to discuss with your doctor and ask for a referral. Unlike other talking therapies, CBT focuses on the present rather than discussing the past, and it works on the idea that physical actions as well as thoughts and feelings are all interconnected. By breaking down your problems into their separate parts and then discussing each separately, you can figure out how to turn around negative thoughts and behaviours and it can really help you deal with issues that you might be finding overwhelming. The great thing about CBT, and another way it differs from other talking therapies, is that you are then equipped to deal with future problems as they arise. As with all talking therapies, there can be some disadvantages, but you will be able to talk through all of these and any additional concerns with your therapist.

4

PCOS (Polycystic ovary syndrome)

What is PCOS?

PCOS is the most common hormone-driven condition in women and those assigned female at birth, affecting up to a quarter of women of reproductive age, meaning that one in every four women may have the condition, and it is the number one cause of subfertility in that population group. Up to 80% of women with anovulatory infertility (infertility caused by the ovaries not releasing an egg during the menstrual cycle) are thought to have PCOS,[1] which means that a high percentage of women turning to fertility treatment to help them conceive have the condition.

To be diagnosed with PCOS under the **Rotterdam criteria** – the internationally agreed diagnostic guide – a woman should have two or more of the following symptoms:

1. An irregular or absent menstrual cycle.
2. Clinical or blood work signs of high levels of androgens. Clinical signs include excess body and facial hair, hair loss or thinning hair on the head, and acne.
3. Polycystic ovaries diagnosed via an ultrasound.

Contrary to the name, the 'cysts' seen on polycystic ovaries are not actually cysts at all, but fluid-filled sacs, or follicles, which develop on the ovaries during the menstrual cycle and interfere with normal ovulation because the sacs are often unable to release an egg. Not all women with PCOS will have these though and their absence does not mean the absence of the condition. This part of the diagnostic criteria is also not suitable for use with young women within eight years of starting their period. This is because there is a risk of over-diagnosis as many young women will have ovaries with multiple small follicles during this time. This may lead to clinicians diagnosing them with PCOS when actually it is a normal part of this developmental stage.

The fact that not all women will have fluid-filled sacs on their ovaries is really important to highlight as many women think that PCOS is a syndrome caused purely by a disorder of the ovaries. This is actually not true. PCOS is an endocrine (hormone) system disorder which affects the function of the ovaries, not a condition of the ovaries themselves, and it also causes general metabolic symptoms. What demonstrates this clearly is the fact that men can be affected by symptoms of PCOS, which may surprise you as the vast majority of people see it as a condition that only affects women.

PCOS was first identified in 1935 as a gynaecological disorder, but understanding of the disease has progressed since then and the more recent discovery that there is a genetic link means that brothers and fathers of women with PCOS can also experience high androgen levels and therefore face the same metabolic health risks. This means having an increased risk of type 2 diabetes, obesity and heart disease. So, we should not be thinking of PCOS as a women-only condition. Men with a female history of PCOS in their family should be monitored for these chronic diseases that can also impact fertility.

Understanding the endocrine system

I'll briefly explain what the endocrine system is as it is important to understand this. It is basically a collection of organs and tissues which secrete hormones. These then act as chemical messengers when they are released into the bloodstream. They travel to different organs and when they get there they have metabolic or reproductive effects. These hormones are released all over the body, including from the brain, thyroid gland, testicles, ovaries, pancreas and adrenal glands. If there is an imbalance of hormones in the body, symptoms can develop, including weight gain, excess body hair, skin problems, hair loss, fatigue, depression, disruptions to the menstrual cycle and insulin resistance. Insulin resistance results in higher levels of insulin in the bloodstream (see below). Higher levels of circulating insulin – the hormone that regulates glucose levels in the bloodstream among other things – mean higher androgen levels. So, things become a bit of a vicious circle.

As well as the physical conditions associated with PCOS, it can also have profound psychological consequences. This is a result of both the symptoms and the poor understanding by others, especially if a woman experiences frequent, severe acne, hair loss and/ or excess body hair. These consequences include low self-esteem, poor body image, anxiety and problems sleeping. Depression has also been shown to be significantly higher in women with PCOS, with women who have a BMI over 30 experiencing higher rates of depression than those who are a healthy weight.[2]

Pregnancy complications can also be higher in women with PCOS. These include a significantly increased risk of developing gestational diabetes, as well as an increased risk of high blood pressure, pre-eclampsia, smaller birth-weight babies, and having to have a caesarian section delivery.[3]

PCOS is a complex condition, and the cause is not fully understood. We know there is a combination of lifestyle and genetic factors involved and it is chronic, meaning there is no cure. However, making positive dietary and lifestyle changes can help to manage symptoms. One reason for this is that it enables the body's tissues to use insulin more effectively and, as insulin levels drop, so do androgen levels. This is why it is so important to seek help if you have PCOS because symptoms really can be improved with the right support and guidance.

Hyperandrogenism explained

Androgens are often referred to as 'male sex hormones' but actually this is unhelpful and also inaccurate. Yes, males may make more of them, with testosterone being the most common type, but females also make androgens. Referring to them as male sex hormones in PCOS only adds to the stigma attached to the condition. In addition, for the many women psychologically affected by their condition, telling them they have excess male sex hormones is only going to fuel their anxiety and poor body image.

Higher circulating levels of androgens is one of the main diagnostic criteria for PCOS and is thought to affect up to 80% of patients with the condition.[4] This is why so many women with PCOS experience infertility as it causes disruptions to the menstrual cycle. Many may not seek help out of embarrassment or the stigma attached to their symptoms, and I have had women telling me about previous negative experiences with a healthcare provider which may have put them off seeking further help. This makes me sad and also really angry because this should never be the case and I would urge you if you are struggling with symptoms of PCOS to find an empathetic medical professional who will give you the support you deserve.

What is insulin resistance?

Insulin is a hormone produced by the pancreas and its main job, as mentioned above, is to regulate the amount of glucose in the blood. When we eat, the carbohydrates in our food are broken down into glucose (a type of sugar). This is then absorbed in our small intestine and released into our bloodstream. It is insulin's job to help remove this glucose from our bloodstream and get it into our muscle and fat cells, where it can be used for energy. You can think of insulin as a key as it unlocks our cells to allow the glucose in.

Problems start to happen when insulin stops acting in the way it should because the body is less responsive to it. This is called insulin resistance and, whereas the incidence in the general population is around 10-25%, in women with PCOS it may be as high as 95%.[5] Initially the pancreas will produce more insulin to help 'unlock' the cells (this is called hyperinsulinaemia) but this is only a short-term solution and eventually, without any changes in diet/lifestyle, the person with insulin resistance will develop type 2 diabetes.

Insulin resistance is more severe in women with obesity, but it does still occur in women of a healthy weight and therefore diet and lifestyle adaptions in order to address insulin resistance are key. This is so important for women trying to conceive, not only to help them increase their chances but also to reduce the risk of developing gestational diabetes. Visceral body fat, which is the fat stored within the abdominal cavity and that can surround several organs, increases the risk of insulin resistance and can occur in women who may have what is considered a healthy BMI (body mass index – see page 69). These individuals are often referred to as 'skinny fat', not a term I agree with but so-called because they may appear slim on the outside but have excess fat inside that cannot be seen with the naked eye. This is one reason why BMI alone is a poor indicator of health and should always be used alongside other measurements, such as waist circumference.

Women with higher circulating androgens seem to be at increased risk of insulin resistance, but it is unclear whether the increased hormones result from insulin resistance, whether insulin resistance occurs as a result of higher androgen levels, or whether they both occur independently. The general thinking though is that insulin resistance is the primary problem and hyperandrogenism is secondary. This is because, unlike other tissues and organs in the body, the ovaries remain insulin sensitive, so insulin resistance does not occur there. When the pancreas releases more insulin in response to insulin resistance in other parts of the body, the ovaries release androgens and levels of SHBG decrease, which then leads to higher circulating levels of androgens. It can also lead to lower levels of luteinising hormone (LH) and follicle stimulating hormone (FSH), which can lead to infrequent ovulation or prevent it altogether.

PCOS and vitamin D

Women with PCOS are also more likely to be deficient in vitamin D, having up to an 85% chance of being deficient compared with up to a 48% chance in the general population.[6] However, we cannot say that deficiency causes these conditions. What we can say is that vitamin D appears to play an important part in PCOS in that supplementation has been associated with an increased number of dominant follicles. It has also been suggested that supplementing vitamin D along with the diabetes drug, metformin (which may be used as part of treatment for PCOS), may regulate menstrual cycles better than if metformin is given alone.[7] Another study highlighted the important role of vitamin D when the authors found that women with PCOS who were infertile had lower vitamin D levels than the women with PCOS who were fertile.[6] This suggests the vitamin is important for ovulatory function and fertility in women with the hormone-driven condition.

Are women with PCOS more prone to carrying excess weight?

This is a question I am often asked but actually it isn't something we know a huge amount about and studies have shown conflicting outcomes. It is not clear therefore whether obesity is caused by PCOS, or whether it is a factor in its development.

As I have said, not all women with PCOS are above what is considered the healthy weight range, but many are and unfortunately this may be set to rise alongside the increasing rates of obesity in the general population. For these women, losing as little as 5-10% of body weight has been shown to benefit reproductive and physical health, including the restoration of a normal menstrual cycle, achieving pregnancy and a reduction in miscarriage rates. It can also reduce the risk of type 2 diabetes and metabolic syndrome common in women with PCOS.[8] Metabolic syndrome is a cluster of conditions that can increase the risk of heart disease, stroke and type 2 diabetes and includes high blood pressure, high blood glucose levels, high cholesterol and having excess fat around the middle.

However, this topic needs to be approached carefully as weight is a very sensitive issue and unfortunately many healthcare providers approach it in the wrong way. I have had patients telling me they visited their doctor to discuss their symptoms and were told out of the blue and very insensitively that they needed to lose weight when they were not even aware the topic was going to be broached. This then resulted in a negative experience because they did not feel in control of the situation, and in some situations felt humiliated. They then went home feeling they had been dismissed and not taken seriously. To make the situation even worse, some felt as though their doctor had placed the blame on them for being overweight and that help would not be available until they had managed to lose weight. The obvious aside, this judgmental approach is so counterproductive because someone who is shamed into trying to lose weight will, nine times out of 10, not lose weight.

Even though weight loss has been shown to help manage PCOS symptoms, the focus should not be on weight itself but on improving general health by increasing physical activity, improving diet quality, and being able to access a counselling service if needed. In fact, there are International Guidelines that recognise the importance of approaching PCOS in a holistic way, with the focus being on education, self-empowerment and psychological and physical wellbeing.[7]

Many women with PCOS not only carry the stigma associated with the condition itself but also that attached to being overweight or obese. There is still very much the attitude, often fueled by the media, that obesity is simply a result of someone eating too much and not doing any exercise. The truth is it is far more complicated than that. There are often many factors involved, including past and present trauma, disordered eating and underlying medical conditions, and if these factors are not addressed, the person will not get the help they need.

One study looking into whether women with PCOS have a genetic predisposition for overweight or obesity found no such link when looking specifically at genes associated with BMI.[9] The authors concluded weight gain in women with PCOS was likely due to a combination of other genetic factors and environmental factors. Women with PCOS reported higher energy intakes and more sedentary lifestyles than women without PCOS. Other factors that meant weight gain was more likely included the consumption of higher amounts of refined carbohydrates, as well as smoking, ethnicity, alcohol intake and employment type.

However, a more recent study had a different outcome.[10] Women from a variety of cultural backgrounds took part, including South and East Asians, Europeans and Australian Aboriginals, and the role of dietary intake and activity levels in PCOS was assessed. Macro- and micronutrient intakes were also examined to observe any associations between these and symptoms of PCOS, including insulin resistance, obesity and hyperandrogenism.

The results of the study showed that, despite significant differences in weight and BMI, calorie intake and exercise levels did not differ significantly between women with PCOS and women without. This goes against the suggestion that women with PCOS may consume excess calories and exercise less than women without PCOS.

Lower fibre, vitamin A and magnesium intakes and higher refined carbohydrate intakes were seen in women with PCOS compared with those without and were all associated with insulin resistance in these women. Lower fibre was also associated with higher total cholesterol and triglyceride levels.

Lower fibre being associated with an increased risk of insulin resistance is not surprising. Fibre slows down the absorption of glucose and can therefore help to regulate blood glucose levels, as well as aiding weight management. One reason for this is that some of the energy contained in high-fibre foods becomes a component of your poo rather than being absorbed. The women with PCOS in the study only consumed on average 19.6 g of fibre per day which is similar to the UK's average fibre intake and much lower than the recommended intake of 30 g per day. This demonstrates the importance of increasing fibre intakes as part of dietary management of PCOS, as well as ensuring adequate intakes of micronutrients, including vitamin A and magnesium.

How does excess weight affect PCOS?

We now know the effects of obesity on insulin resistance and the increased production of androgens, but high levels of insulin can also result in further weight gain as it is an appetite stimulant. Many women with PCOS will report regular cravings for refined carbohydrate-rich foods, such as sugar-sweetened drinks, cakes, biscuits and 'stodgy' foods, such as white pasta and bread. This means that vicious circle comes back so it is really important to implement changes that can help reduce insulin resistance and thereby reduce the risk of developing type 2 diabetes, as well as improving fertility. An additional problem is that high levels of glucose in the blood act as a source of oxidative stress and we know this directly impairs fertility by damaging egg and sperm cells.

Wider health implications

An ongoing study, the Apple Women's Health Study, which started in 2019, has highlighted the wider health impacts of PCOS. The study, which currently has around 37,000 participants (anyone can enroll in the study at any time) has shown that women with PCOS have a higher prevalence of conditions that can negatively affect heart health. This includes them being almost four times more likely to have pre-diabetic conditions, three times more likely to have type 2 diabetes, 1.7 times more likely to have high blood pressure and high cholesterol, and just over 25% more likely to have obesity than women without PCOS.[11] This preliminary data showed just how important it was for women with PCOS to make positive nutrition and lifestyle changes, not just to improve their fertility but also to reduce their risk of developing chronic disease.

So, what is the solution?

The key is focusing on healthy lifestyle changes that will result in gradual, sustainable weight loss. The problem is there are lots of crash diets out there, promising to deliver rapid weight loss, and this can be very tempting. If women seek support and follow a weight loss programme purely aimed at calorie restriction, although weight loss may initially happen, most of the weight is likely to be regained within one year. We know that on the whole, 'diets' do not work as the basis of every weight loss diet is restriction. Certain foods may be demonised, some meals may be replaced by shakes, and often calorie restriction is significant, leading to hunger, despondency and ultimately a return to previous eating habits. Plus, who wants to have to step on the scales in front of a group of strangers and either be applauded for weight loss or commiserated with for not having lost weight? I have heard women talking to each other in changing rooms before their weekly weigh-in who have skipped breakfast and lunch and have minimised their fluid intake to optimise their chances of the scales showing a loss. That is no way to live your life.

An approach like this towards food encourages disordered eating and can mean a life-long negative body image as well as a poor relationship with food. A predominantly whole food plant-based diet, on the other hand, is not a 'diet' in the traditional sense but rather a dietary pattern that, although it minimises or eliminates animal products, focuses on what you can add into your diet to make every meal colourful, tasty and satisfying. It focuses on including a huge variety of different grains, vegetables, fruit, nuts, seeds and legumes; after all, there are around 2000 plant species in the world that are cultivated by humans for food. That is incredible, right? The choice is almost endless!

The importance of exercise

Exercising is important for all aspects of health, but for women with insulin resistance it has two extra benefits:

1. It can help your muscles take up glucose: When you sit down for long periods of time, your large muscles relax and this means they do not take up much glucose from your blood. If they are already struggling to do this because they are resistant to the actions of insulin, this will not help and will increase your risk of developing type 2 diabetes. The best thing you can do is to keep moving, even if that means standing up from your desk every hour and walking around to flex your large muscles. I always use my fitness watch to make sure I get up during a day's writing. Just walking around or doing a few star jumps, stretches or squats, can help get those muscles activated and the blood flowing.

2. It can lower blood glucose levels after eating: Doing some form of movement after a meal can help keep blood glucose levels under control as it improves the way your body uses

insulin. We know levels reach their peak about 90 minutes after eating, so doing some form of movement/exercise about half an hour after you eat can be really beneficial. I'm not talking about going for a run or doing strenuous exercise as this will likely make you feel sick, or make symptoms of reflux worse if you suffer from those. Just choosing to iron a pile of clothes after your evening meal, or going for a walk around the block, will help. Remember that if you are not used to exercising and are planning to start, it is always a good idea to get a check up with your GP to make sure that it is safe to do so.

Inositols and improved PCOS parameters

Myo-inositol (MI) is a carbohydrate made in the body but it is also found in whole foods such as fruit, grain, nuts and legumes. It is involved in many functions in the body, including cell growth and survival, bone formation, the development and function of peripheral nerves (the nerves outside of the brain and spinal cord) and reproduction.[12]

MI is the most commonly known inositol and is thought to have a beneficial effect on various parameters in PCOS, including hormone regulation, insulin resistance and improved ovulatory function. It is also essential for the brain and for normal ovary function. Another inositol, D-chiro-inositol (DCI), is also involved in the insulin pathway but in a different way to MI. MI acts to increase the uptake of glucose from the blood into the cells, whereas DCI is involved in the formation of glycogen.[13] Glycogen is the stored form of glucose to be used by the body when energy levels are low. For example, when a long distance runner eats a big bowl of porridge for breakfast, they will use the glucose the body gets from that meal to fuel the first part of their run. When they have used all the glucose, their body will turn to its glucose stores, glycogen. When these are needed, the body will quickly convert it back into glucose to be used for energy. When glycogen stores run out, the body will eventually start to break down muscle unless it gets more glucose. This is why endurance runners often drink sports drinks or take carbohydrate gels during training and racing.

A combination of both MI and DCI may result in better outcomes because they can improve insulin sensitivity in the liver and tissues where glycogen is stored, and also increase MI levels in the ovaries, meaning better FSH sensitivity and oocyte quality.[13]

Due to their beneficial effects on insulin resistance and hormone regulation, inositol supplements are commonly used as a therapeutic treatment for women with PCOS, and have been shown to reduce the severity of excess body and/or facial hair, as well as reduce levels of testosterone and LDL cholesterol,[12] which is the type associated with an increased risk of heart disease and stroke. Other benefits may include an increase in SHBG,[14] which is important as this protein binds with testosterone and prevents it from circulating, thereby reducing the symptoms associated with high circulating androgens.

Inositols are generally deemed to be safe but I would always advise you to speak with your doctor if this is something you would like to explore.

5

Endometriosis

What is endometriosis?

Endometriosis is a chronic, inflammatory, oestrogen-dependent disease that affects 10-15% of women of reproductive age.[1] This means that around 1.5 million women and those assigned female at birth are living with the condition. There is the real risk of a significant impact on quality of life because, as it can take on average eight years to diagnose, women are living with chronic pain and fatigue that can have negative effects on relationships, and can also result in infertility. Endometriosis is thought to affect up to 22% of women of reproductive age, but in women with irregular or absent periods it is much higher, with up to 60% affected.[1]

The condition arises where cells similar to those that line a woman's uterus, which grow and bleed with each menstrual cycle, are found elsewhere in the body. The most common place for cells to grow is in the pelvic cavity, but they have also been found in the intestine, bladder, liver, kidney and nasal cavity, on caesarian scars, and even in rare cases in the lungs and brain. These cells respond to each menstrual cycle and bleed but, unlike those in the womb which are shed as a woman's monthly period, the cells that grow elsewhere in the body have nowhere to go and so become inflamed. This results in pain and the formation of scar tissue, which can then lead to pelvic pain, bowel and bladder symptoms, painful and/ or heavy periods, painful sex and infertility. As symptoms can be very similar to irritable bowel syndrome (IBS), diagnosis can be delayed by women being referred to see a gut specialist rather than a gynaecologist, so it is really important when you first see your GP that you give as much information as you can. Writing down a list of all your symptoms means that you are less likely to forget to mention something relevant, and it would be helpful to take along a pain and symptom diary. I would suggest for a week before your appointment (longer if you can) write down when you experience pain and where, how painful it is on a scale of 0-10 and any other symptoms that you get throughout the day or night.

I can really empathise with anyone who has experienced the pain of endometriosis during their period. It really can be excruciating. When it flared up for me during my degree there were days when I couldn't even sit up straight, let alone walk and get on with my daily activities. The only way I could manage the pain was to lie curled up in a ball in bed or on the sofa with a hot water bottle. I don't think anyone who hasn't experienced this has any idea how debilitating it can be.

The only way to get a definitive diagnosis of endometriosis unfortunately is by an operation called a laparoscopy. This is when a camera is inserted into the pelvis via a small incision near the belly button and the surgeon then uses the camera to have a look to see if there are any signs of the disease. The problem with this is it's a pretty invasive procedure, with the need for a general anaesthetic, and even if the patches of endometriosis are removed, the recurrence rate is fairly high. Although some studies have looked at diet as an alternative way of managing endometriosis, there are still no set dietary guidelines for endometriosis management. There is, however, growing evidence that reducing/avoiding meat and building the diet around high-fibre plant foods may help manage symptoms.

Animal foods and risk

Oxidative stress seems to be one factor in the development of endometriosis as it causes an inflammatory response in the peritoneal fluid.[2] This is the fluid that is made in the abdominal cavity to act as a lubricant and covers most of the organs in that space. We know that haem iron in animal foods acts as a source of oxidative stress, so minimising or eliminating this from your diet makes sense to reduce the risk of this inflammatory response.

Standard Western diets high in animal foods and processed meat, in particular ham, beef and other kinds of red meat, are associated with a significantly higher risk of developing endo-metriosis.[3] Poultry has also been shown to increase the risk but not as significantly as red meat. Dairy has not been consistently shown to increase the risk and has actually been shown in a recent review to reduce the risk of developing endometriosis for women regularly consuming cheese and milk. Butter on the other hand may increase the risk.[4] One explanation may be the vitamin D and calcium content in dairy. Vitamin D has been shown to regu-late immune function and, as women with endometriosis display immune changes, vitamin D may be beneficial. It has been shown that women with higher blood levels of vitamin D have a 24% lower risk of endometriosis than women with the lowest blood levels, and adequate calcium and vitamin D intakes from food are associated with a lower risk.[5] I am not going to tell you then that dairy is a risk factor for endometriosis. What I will say is that you can easily meet your calcium and vitamin D requirements without dairy. As long as you are meeting your needs, the effects will likely be the same as if you consumed these nutrients from dairy, especially as the cal-cium from fortified products has the same absorption rate as that from dairy.

Benefits of plant foods

Whole plant foods can have positive effects on oestrogen levels and can increase those carrier proteins, SHBGs. The oestrogen-lower-ing effects happen via two main mechanisms. Whole plant foods are high in fibre and we know fibre binds with excess hormones to remove them from your body. The insulin-lowering effects of fibre are also significant because higher levels of insulin increase oestrogen and endometrial cell production – two great reasons to pack that fibre in.

Fruit is associated with a reduced risk of endometriosis, particularly citrus fruit, and this may be due to their beta-cryptoxanthin content (a carotenoid with antioxidant properties) as well as the fact they are high in vitamin C.[6] The growth of endometrial tissue in the peritoneal cavity may be influenced by oxidative stress and, as vitamin C acts as an antioxidant to neutralise the damage caused by oxidative stress, this may partly explain the association. Data from the Nurses Health Study II show that vitamin C from food and supplements combined, or from supplements alone, does not have the same association, meaning there may be a threshold to the beneficial effects of vitamin C. When you consider the side effects of high doses of vitamin C (see page 151), this makes sense as it is important to remember that more isn't always better.

Interestingly, high intakes of cruciferous vegetables have been shown to be associated with an increased risk of endometriosis,[6] but when you look into why this may be, it is likely linked to many of them being high in certain carbohydrates, known as FODMAPs, that can exacerbate symptoms of IBS, and this can be difficult to differentiate from chronic abdominal pain caused by endometriosis. These vegetables include cauliflower, broccoli, cabbage and Brussels sprouts.

This association between cruciferous vegetables and a higher risk of endometriosis is likely due to increased abdominal pain and other GI symptoms that subsequently lead to a diagnosis of endometriosis, rather than the vegetables themselves increasing the risk. When we look at the components of these vegetables, they are packed with fibre, phytonutrients, vitamins and minerals that are known to reduce the risk of many chronic conditions as well as helping to optimise fertility. Rather than avoiding them, if you notice eating them makes you feel very bloated or causes unwanted wind or means that you are dashing to the loo with some urgency, you can try including them initially in small quantities. You can then increase your portion sizes until you find a level you can tolerate. This could mean initially having just 1-2 tbsp of one of these vegetables at a time, and increasing every three to four days by 1-2 tbsp. If you really struggle with GI symptoms though, I would advise asking your GP/doctor for a referral to see a specialist dietitian who can help you.

Omega-3 fats have been associated with a lower risk of endometriosis,[7] so it may be beneficial to pay extra attention to these fats and to take a daily supplement, as discussed in Chapter 20.

Future study

A clinical trial is currently taking place looking at women aged between 18 and 51 years with a clinical diagnosis of endometriosis. The researchers are giving one group Flexofytol, a capsule containing 42 mg of curcumin twice a day, for four months in place of the participants' usual pain-relieving medications. The primary outcome measure will be change in the average pain score from baseline (the start of the study) to four months (the duration of the study). There will also be a number of secondary outcomes, including changes in the number of days with pain, quality of life and painful intercourse, urination and bowel movements.

The trial is the 'gold standard' of trials, being randomised, double-blind and placebo controlled. This means that the participants are assigned randomly to either the intervention or placebo group (these will be given a substitute for the curcumin which has no known ingredients that will affect the outcome), and neither they nor the investigators will know to which group they have been allocated. This reduces the risk of the outcome being affected by either the patients' or investigator's expectations.

We already have data showing that administering curcumin via capsules, ointment or fresh/ground turmeric can exert anti-viral, antioxidant, anti-inflammatory and anti-tumour effects. We also have more recent data showing that it can improve pain, including in sciatica, chemotherapy-induced nerve inflammation,[8] and arthritic knee pain in older adults.[9] The outcome of this trial is much anticipated as it could potentially provide evidence of a simple dietary therapy which may offer relief to many women experiencing chronic endometrial pain, without the need for long-term pain-relieving medications.

The benefits of exercise

Although there is a lack of well-designed studies looking at the benefits of exercise for endometriosis, we do know that exercise appears to be beneficial for conditions that involve inflammatory processes. This is partly because it increases various substances, called cytokines, that are released by the immune system which have anti-inflammatory properties.

A review suggests a number of positive benefits from exercising, including up to a 65% lower risk of developing endometriosis with regular exercise of a minimum of two hours a week.[1] It was also suggested that regular daily exercise is a more effective form of pain relief than taking painkillers and without any of the potential side effects. These are all positive findings; however, we need controlled, randomised trials to really get to the bottom of how effective exercise is in terms of reducing endometriosis risk and managing its associated symptoms.

A more recent review looking at whether exercise can help manage symptoms of endometriosis concluded that, although firm recommendations can't be made based on the quality of existing studies, women should be advised that there are potential benefits.[10]

We know that exercise is beneficial to general health for many reasons. It can help us build strong bones and muscle when a combination of strength and cardio exercise is performed regularly, and it can help to improve mood because it stimulates the release of happy hormones from our brains. It helps to keep our cardiovascular system healthy, increases insulin sensitivity thereby reducing insulin resistance, and lowers blood pressure and cholesterol when combined with positive dietary changes. It can help to improve energy levels, concentration and sleep (as long as you are not doing intense exercise within a few hours of going to bed).

How much exercise should you be aiming for?

The UK guidelines recommend aiming for a minimum of 150 minutes of moderate exercise a week, but the important thing is to start a regimen that suits you initially and listen to your body. If you find that on some days you are in a lot of pain, don't force yourself into exercising as this may make you feel worse. Conversely, if your pain is manageable, exercise may make you feel better. On bad days, try to still move your body as much as you can by going for a few short, gentle walks, or doing some gentle stretches, although I understand that on some of those days the pain can be too bad even to stand up straight, let alone walk. On the days when you don't experience as much pain, aim to make those your moderate sessions where you increase the pace and get your heart rate up. By doing this, you should be able eventually to get up to those 150 minutes. You may also identify certain exercises that make your pain symptoms worse, such as those that involve impact like running. If you want to run but this happens, then just take it back down to a fast walk and gently try to build up on the days when your pain levels are low.

The amount of time you exercise for is also entirely up to you. You may prefer to do 30-60 minutes at a time, or break it down into smaller 10-15-minute sessions, or even just five minutes at a time.

And remember that exercising doesn't mean having to join a gym or paying for classes; it can be anything you want it to be as long as your body is moving and your heart rate is elevated. Dancing around your kitchen, going for a walk, swimming or doing sets of body weight exercises at home all count. I would also advise you to have active rest days, which means that on the days you are not exercising, try to avoid sitting for long periods and still aim to go outside for a short walk.

6

Inequalities in fertility care

I want to start this chapter by saying that the issue of inequalities in fertility care, especially those relating to race and ethnicity, is a hugely important and complex topic. I have done my best to highlight the key areas to increase awareness of the inequalities that may be affecting you but it is by no means exhaustive. I feel very strongly that all healthcare professionals (HCPs) need to and should be aware of these issues and educate themselves so that things can start to improve. This topic really is a book in itself and I would encourage you to do further reading, especially if these issues do not affect you directly but you would like to fully appreciate what ethnic minority groups in the UK, and people of colour worldwide, have had to endure historically and to this day.

As with all areas of health and any other area in life, inclusivity is vital and ethnicity and race must be a part of the conversation. It is important to highlight that even now there continue to be inequalities in access to healthcare. Unfortunately, some groups can have a much tougher time when it comes to accessing medical treatment and care relating to subfertility, as well as encountering bias from those in charge of their care.

What I didn't realise until I started researching this chapter is that Asian or South Asian women account for just over 4% of those living with subfertility in the UK. However, their ethnicity is suggested as a risk factor itself for early ovarian aging and poorer IVF outcomes in many studies rather than looking at other contributing factors.[1] These studies have been criticised for a number of reasons, including small numbers of participants and selection bias. This means the group selected for the study is not representative of the target population. Missing data is also an issue as it means the results are inaccurate.

The first study to compare White women with Indian women born in Britain undergoing IVF treatment was in 1995.[2] Differences were found between groups in response to ovarian stimulation and rates of miscarriage. This led the authors to conclude that Indian women had poorer IVF outcomes than White women, or in their words 'Indians performed worse than Whites.' I felt uncomfortable when I read this and also when I typed it, but I wanted to draw attention to the language chosen by the authors, which is discriminatory in itself. The authors of the study cited a report from India as the reason behind investigating further in their own study. This report had been published in a journal and was written by a team from a research centre and hospital in Mumbai, India, who had expressed their surprise at their low IVF success rates. They wrote that almost one third of their patients did not respond to ovarian stimulation and as a result their pregnancy rates were low compared with other centres worldwide. The authors of the report did explain that the reasons for this were likely due to their lack of experience in IVF and their new laboratory set-up, and that actually their results were comparable to the success rates of other clinics that were practising new IVF techniques at the time. Despite this, their results were explained by research groups in the UK as showing clear differences between White and Indian women, with Indian women having poorer IVF outcomes. To me, this shows the limitations of the study were ignored by research groups in the UK who formed their own discriminatory conclusions and encouraged this to continue to filter through the scientific community.

Historically, the majority of fertility studies have focused on women going through fertility treatment and as this has only included small numbers of ethnic minority populations, the exploration of ethnic inequalities in fertility has been limited.

The under-representation of ethnic and religious minority groups in European studies on infertility means that HCPs may have a lack of understanding of these patients' experiences of their infertility journey and/or treatment, and there is a lack of guidance aimed at supporting these patient groups. Some reasons for this lack of inclusivity may include barriers to accessing healthcare, which include stigma attached to infertility in the patient's cultural setting, language barriers, lack of access to healthcare systems where research takes place, and distrust in the healthcare system as a result of previous negative experiences, meaning they do not want to take part in research. These are important factors to understand as it means there are far wider reasons for poorer fertility outcomes than just ethnicity.[1]

What other factors could be present?

Socioeconomic status

Socioeconomic status is a hugely important point as fertility treatment is expensive. A recent study looking at disparities in access to fertility care in the US found that Black and Hispanic participants were twice as likely to report cost of treatment and/or medication as a barrier to accessing fertility treatment than White and Asian participants.[3] The participants were also asked to list other factors that made it more difficult to access fertility treatment, and race was given as a factor by 14.7% of Black participants compared with 0% of White and just over 5% of Hispanic and Asian participants. This shows that the White participants had never considered race to be a barrier and this is really meaningful.

Distrust of medical services

This is especially relevant within the Black community and was highlighted in a recent report in the *Lancet*, a highly respected medical journal.[4] This distrust stems from historical racism within the medical system, which began with the treatment of Black people between 1619 (when the first enslaved people were brought to the British Colony of Virginia) and 1865 (when the last enslaved Black person was emancipated in the US). This included violent medical treatment and forced experimentation. Medical schools would also use freshly buried and disinterred bodies of Black people for dissection, depriving them of a dignified and peaceful burial. What made this awful practice worse was these schools employed Black men to do the job of retrieving bodies for this purpose as they felt a White person would be too conspicuous walking into a cemetery. Shockingly, in 1907 compulsory sterilisation laws in the US were established. This led to the forced sterilisation of almost 60,000 people. The practice involving Black women continued until into the 1980s even though the law was overturned in the 60s and 70s. People of colour made up the vast majority of those being forced into sterilisation, with African–American people making up nearly 5000 of the 8000 sterilised in North Carolina. There are many other awful practices that have taken place in the not-so-distant past and the shadows of these are still very present today. These include the forced sterilisation of hundreds of thousands of men and women of reproductive age in Nazi Germany with genetic, mental and physical health disorders, and the treatment of unmarried women throughout the UK as recently as the 1970s who were forced to give up their babies for adoption.

A recent review by the NHS Race and Health Observatory highlights ethnic inequalities in maternal and neonatal healthcare in England, with poor communication cited frequently as a major reason for suboptimal care.[5] For women whose first language is not English, the lack of accessibility to high quality interpreters for medical appointments is a common theme. However, even for British-born ethnic minority women and migrant women who can speak English, communication can also be compromised. Many explanations for this are given, including lack of sensitivity, poor listening skills by the healthcare provider and poor understanding of cultural differences and failure to address this. Women reported feeling disrespected, stereotyped and discriminated against which resulted in distrust, feeling poorly cared for and less willing to access and engage with services. The report highlighted one study looking at ethnic inequalities in neonatal (newborn) care, where a high proportion of Asian babies were mistakenly admitted to neo-natal wards for treatment of jaundice. The report recommends the need for serious commitment by NHS services in England to tackle both racist attitudes and racist behaviours by staff and address the structures within the NHS itself that discriminate against eth-nic-minority women and their babies.

Differences in fertility treatment outcomes

For those accessing fertility treatment, a HFEA report in 2018 revealed that live birth rates from IVF varied by patient ethnic group.[6] Higher birth rates were recorded for White and Mixed ethnicity patients, whereas Black patients (especially those identi-fying as Black African) and Asian (especially South Asian) patients had lower birth rates. The reasons for these differences are not clear, but there may be a number of different factors involved. These include socioeconomic-related underlying conditions, such as excess weight, as this can reduce the ovarian response to the drugs used to stimulate them during treatment. Another reason may include the higher incidence of fibroids among Black women which are associated with poorer IVF outcomes.

Learning from personal experiences

A really interesting, recent study recruited nine ethnic minority women living in Wales to attend a one-day drawing workshop with the aim of enabling them to express their experiences and views of infertility, as well as their fertility care needs.[7] The ethnic backgrounds of the women were South Asian Muslim, Sub-Saharan African Christian, North African Muslim and British Muslim. The workshop involved the women choosing an infertility-related drawing they felt most connected with and drawing themselves thinking or talking about infertility. They were asked to draw visual metaphors for their infertility experience. For example, 'if infertility was a drawing or an animal what would it be?' There was also a free drawing session, and then finally a group sharing session. Many themes were identified as a result of these tasks, but I wish to focus on three: what the paper calls the 'social burden of infertility', the community, and healthcare experiences.

The social burden of infertility

Most of the women had experienced difficult and stressful social interactions with members of their husband's close family around the subject of parenthood. They would have frequent questions relating to either the absence of children or the fact they only had one child. These conversations would continue among their friends and other members of the community, with people often saying insensitive things or constantly asking when they are going to become pregnant. Some even encouraged their partners to leave and find a woman who could provide them with children. These comments and questions were then likely to make the women withdraw from their social circles and made them feel isolated from their partner, family and friends. When asked to draw visual metaphors, the women chose walls, a prison or a valley, depicting how shut off, trapped and isolated they were by these questions and comments. Metaphors can be very powerful and choosing a prison to explain how they were feeling is profound. I think we take for granted just how supported we are most of the time if we are lucky to have accessible healthcare and nurturing relationships and are free to talk about subfertility without feeling as though it is something shameful to keep hidden.

The community

The women described the traditionalist views of women in their community, with their being seen almost exclusively as mothers. This means that to experience subfertility puts a large social burden on them as the expectation is to have children soon after being married. If this does not happen and subfertility is suspected, the woman will be blamed as male infertility is not spoken about and is seen as a taboo subject. This demonstrates the difficulties in treating male-factor infertility in these communities as they are unlikely to seek help. Suggestions on how to address this have been made in other studies, with one suggesting religious leaders be approached as they may be in a better position to encourage the males within their community to speak out.[1]

Healthcare experience

Positively, the women in the study did not believe themselves to have been discriminated against within the National Health Service (NHS). However, we know from other findings that there is widespread discrimination and racism within the NHS. This does not just affect service users but also staff.[8] Some of the women did comment that they experienced a lack of understanding and even felt ignored by some HCPs who did not empathise with their desire to have more than one child or their reluctance to use donated sperm during fertility treatment. They also reported feeling as though they were not listened to and as a result had been given inappropriate advice. If this hits home for you I would encourage you to educate your HCP so that you are able to be given tailored advice. It is so important to be treated as an individual and if you feel you are not receiving the best care as a result of ignorance it is so important to voice your concerns. Highlighting additional training needs can also help to bring about positive change.

Glossary

Race – defined as a category of people who share certain inherited characteristics, such as skin colour and facial features.

Ethnicity – this is a broader term than race as it categorises people according to their culture and identity. For example, someone may state their race as White and their Ethnicity as Irish, or their race as Black and their Ethnicity as French.

What research tells us about racial and ethnic differences

A recent review of 37 studies looking at racial and ethnic disparities in fertility care raised many important issues.[9]

There was found to be a higher prevalence of uterine fibroids in Black women, with a 25.5% prevalence compared to White women in whom there was a 6.9% prevalence. Fibroids can result in subfertility, can also be debilitating and can result in poorer IVF outcomes. It is important for you to be aware of the symptoms of fibroids so you can discuss these with your doctor if you have any concerns. These include heavy periods or prolonged periods lasting more than seven days, abdominal pain, lower back pain, urinating more frequently, pain or discomfort during sex and constipation.

The review also highlighted a national population-based survey called the National Survey of Family Growth (NSFG). This has been sent out to hundreds of thousands of people in America since 1973 to gather information on infertility, pregnancy, men and women's health, and also family life, marriage and divorce.

Data for between 1982 and 2002 were analysed and showed large disparities in accessibility to fertility services between ethnic and racial groups. Each ethnic group other than White was more likely to have infertility than White women but they were also far less likely to access treatment. Black women were 29% less likely to report having received treatment. Data from 2006-2010 also showed similar outcomes, with Black and Hispanic women being far less likely to access fertility treatment after being diagnosed with infertility.

More recently, data up to 2013 has been analysed and more ethnic groups added, including Indigenous American women. Again, it was found that Black women had a greater prevalence of infertility but were 47% less likely to access fertility services than White women, showing the problem is getting worse not better. There were initially differences between Hispanic and Indigenous American women compared to White women but after adjustments these were not significant.

The continuous theme of Black women not accessing fertility treatment is relevant as not only are they at higher risk of fibroids which can affect fertility, but they have also been shown to be at a higher risk of miscarriage. A recent report in the *Lancet* suggested that Black women have a 43% higher risk of suffering a miscarriage than White women.[10] This is a really significant percentage and clearly highlights how important it is to make prenatal care, not just fertility care, accessible for all.

The review also found ovarian reserves to be 24.4% lower in African-American women aged 24-45 compared with White women, with Latina women's reserves being 37% lower than White women's and Chinese women's 22% lower. As age progressed to 40-45 years, Latina and Chinese women had lower ovarian reserves than African American women, with the greatest decline being among Chinese women. The reasons for this aren't clear and were not suggested in the review, but it may be due to genetics and the possibility of different rates of ovarian aging between ethnic groups. Other factors that may be at play are different dietary patterns and socioeconomic status. Differences in reproductive hormone production could also play a role, but studies are needed to examine these possibilities further.

Another really important area to highlight is that many women, and men of course, unfortunately have to undergo cancer treatment that may affect their fertility and prevent them from having children after their treatment has finished. For these groups there is the option to have fertility preservation treatment (FPT). This means either collecting eggs and sperm and freezing them separately, or fertilising the egg(s) after collecting naturally or via IVF and then freezing the embryos. The review found that FPT counselling was more likely to happen if the patient was of a younger age (between 18 and 25), had a higher level of education, or had expressed their desire to have children at a later date. One study within the review found that out of 31 African-American women, none was offered FPT counselling. Latina women were also found to have decreased access to FPT compared with White women. This disparity may result in certain ethnic and racial groups not accessing FPT prior to cancer treatment and being left infertile after they have fought and recovered from cancer. Clearly this is a tragic situation and more needs to be done to ensure this does not happen.

As you will also read in the next section, although the studies looked at in this review paper consistently identified ethnic/racial differences in accessing fertility treatment, they did not discuss in depth why this is the case. This is important information to highlight because, as the authors discuss, the preconception period is not the only time ethnic/racial disparities are present; they continue into pregnancy and neonatal care. Economic barriers are often cited in literature but it is important to recognise cultural and social barriers also. These include feelings of guilt at not being able to conceive and shame at being labelled 'infertile'. In parts of Africa, a woman will often be named after her first born, for example 'Mama Naima', but if a woman fails to fall pregnant, she is labelled as 'Mama Nobody', and I find this really heartbreaking. Due to the stigma that infertility carries, many women will not seek help because they do not want other people in their community to know they are infertile. Historical views of Black women being seen as highly fertile due to them being forced into pregnancy during slavery may still be prevalent today and may contribute to this stigma.[9]

Trying to conceive if you are LGBTQIA+

The number of LBGTQIA+ people becoming parents is increasing and this is in part due to the wonder that is reproductive technology. However, the majority of research on fertility, as well as on policies, planning and service provision in healthcare, is aimed at heterosexual couples trying to conceive[11] and this growing community are being largely ignored. Even the WHO's definition of infertility is exclusive, failing to take into account those people who would love to become parents but are biologically unable to without help from either sperm donation, surrogates or fertility treatment. There are calls for this definition to be broadened to include all groups of people whose desire is to have children of their own, and I am fully behind this.

Where LGBTQIA+ people are included in research, important information is excluded. Where studies have found that fertility treatment is underused there is no explanation as to why this may be the case but this is a really important area to explore to enable better understanding and change. Such reasons could include discrimination, limited financial resources, patient education focusing on heterosexual couples and negative experiences with healthcare professionals, including shockingly refusal to proceed with treatment.[11]

If we return to the NSFG and data collected between 2002 and 2010, it was shown that there were also differences in availability of fertility treatment between heterosexual White women and lesbian and bisexual women (classed as 'sexual minority' women), with White heterosexual women receiving fertility treatment at almost double the rate (13% vs 7%).[9]

In the UK, access to fertility care remains very much a postcode lottery, meaning that it is dependent on where you live. A national audit published last year highlighted regional differences in IVF funding which are set by local clinical commissioning groups (CCG). Shockingly the audit found that 90% of CCGs do not offer the National Institute for Health and Care Excellence (NICE)-recommended three full cycles of IVF to eligible women under 40, and 74% do not offer one IVF cycle to women aged 40-42. The audit also found that relationship status affected access to fertility treatment, with only 21% of CCGs offering treatment to single women, and 73% offering treatment to same-sex couples. However, proof of infertility is needed before this treatment is offered, meaning these couples have to go through a minimum of six intrauterine insemination (IUI) rounds which they have to fund themselves. This can become extortionately expensive, cripplingly so when each round can cost up to £1600. This is in stark contrast to heterosexual couples who qualify for NHS treatment if they haven't conceived after two years of trying. This is still a long time to wait but there are no financial implications.

This glaring inequality was addressed in the recently published Women's Health Strategy for England which is such a positive step forward because the current treatment of same-sex couples in my eyes is archaic and disgraceful and I was pleased to see the government recognise this. I do hope this will apply to all couples living in the UK and not just England. The pathway in the NHS will include six rounds of funded IUI and then IVF if needed. How quickly this happens though remains to be seen.

The accessibility of reproductive healthcare for all should be a given but we need research focusing on the LBGTQIA+ community to better understand subfertility within this subgroup as well as barriers experienced when accessing fertility care. Research creates an evidence-base and this in turn should lead to policies and patient information being written that are not focused purely on heterosexual individuals and couples but are inclusive of all, creating a fairer and more empathetic fertility care system.

7

The preconception period

The preconception period is any time before you start trying for a baby. However, as many pregnancies are unplanned, taking control of your health as early as possible will ensure that if you do happen to have an unplanned pregnancy, you can feel reassured to know that you have already made positive changes to improve the health of both you and your baby.

Why is the preconception period a crucial time to make diet and lifestyle changes?

For individuals and couples trying to conceive, the preconception period is a crucial time for optimising egg and sperm health, as well as placental development. To create a healthy baby, you need good quality egg and sperm, which means both parents making healthy diet and lifestyle choices. We now know that the choices you make even before you have conceived your baby can increase their likelihood of getting a chronic disease like type 2 diabetes or heart disease later in life. Isn't that incredible? This is commonly known as 'developmental programming' which means if you, for example, smoke, or eat too little or too much, you could cause permanent changes to your future baby's genetic makeup and metabolism, putting their long-term health, and reproductive health, at risk.[1] This is why the earlier you can start to make positive changes the better.

Three months before trying to conceive is usually enough because it takes roughly this long for the egg to mature and the sperm to develop, and it is during this time that you can really influence their quality. When there are known preconception risk factors, such as poor diet quality and/or being under- or overweight, a longer period of time may be needed to enable positive changes to be implemented. This could mean that it is sensible to wait six months, or even a year, before trying to fall pregnant if you need to make significant changes to your nutrition, or are trying to gain/lose weight to help improve your chances and reduce the risk of pregnancy and birth complications. It is also recommended that if you have had bariatric surgery, you should wait either until your weight has stabilised or between three and six months to minimise the risk of micronutrient deficiencies which are common after such surgery.[2] This is important as many micronutrients play such a vital role in reproductive health, and deficiencies could not only affect your chances of conceiving but could impact on the health of the developing foetus if you do fall pregnant. Chapter 13 will discuss these micronutrients in depth.

The bottom line is, the nutritional status of the father not only influences the health of his sperm but also the health of his future offspring. A mother not only influences the health of her eggs but also her ability to maintain a pregnancy, produce a healthy, effective placenta, enable brain and body development of the foetus, and make and produce nutritious breast milk. So, nutrition is key and I hope that by the end of this book you will feel more confident in knowing how to really nourish your bodies with all the good stuff.

Does weight matter?

Weight is a highly emotive topic and unfortunately one that is not always approached sensitively by HCPs.

Overweight or obesity can be defined as an 'accumulation of abnormal or excess fat that may impair health'.[3] It is well documented that being overweight or obese can increase the risk of serious health conditions, such as heart disease, certain cancers, type 2 diabetes and kidney disease. However, the risks of negative effects on both the female and male reproductive systems are also increased, especially with obesity.

Obesity is a global problem, with the prevalence almost tripling since 1975.[3] The World Health Organization (WHO) estimates that almost two billion adults throughout the world were overweight in 2016, with over 650 million of those people being obese (classed as having a body mass index (BMI) of 30 or above).

To calculate your BMI, you need to work out your height in metres, then square it (times it by itself) and divide by your weight in kg. (Alternatively, you can look it up online if you know your height and weight – for example, at www.nhs.uk/live-well/healthy-weight/bmi-calculator/.) For example, a woman who is 1.68 m (2.82 m^2) and weighs 60 kg would have a BMI of 21.3 kg/m^2 '(60 kg divided by 2.82 m^2). This would put her in the healthy weight range for her height. The healthy range used in the NHS is between 18.5 and 24.9. If you fall under this you are classed as underweight and if you fall over this you are classed as overweight. If your BMI is above 30 you are classed as obese.

There are many risks associated with female obesity for fertility and pregnancy, including struggling to conceive, pregnancy complications such as gestational diabetes and pre-eclampsia, large birth-weight babies, stillbirths, congenital abnormalities and an increased risk of maternal death.[4] It has been shown that for every unit increase in BMI over 29, there is a 5% reduced chance of conception among sub fertile women.[5] There are also negative effects on egg quality and implantation during in-vitro fertilisation (IVF). In terms of hormone health, more oestrogen is made in body fat so the higher the percentage of body fat a woman has, the more oestrogen is produced, as well as testosterone, and lower levels of SHBG are common. This leads to hormonal imbalances which can then lead to subfertility.

For men, some studies have shown negative impacts on sperm of being overweight, whereas others have shown that it may be beneficial to be overweight but not obese. A review of 21 studies looking at over 13,000 men attending fertility clinics found that overweight and obese men had a significantly increased risk of having an abnormal sperm count or azoospermia (absence of sperm) when compared with men who were a healthy weight.[6] However, a recent study found that being overweight might increase the chance of conception.[7] They suggest the optimum BMI for women trying to conceive is between 20-23, and for men between 22 and 27. A BMI above 25 puts you in the overweight category so the range in men accounts for being slightly overweight. The authors suggest the best combination for pregnancy success is where the woman is within the healthy BMI range and the man is either within the healthy range or slightly overweight.

So, while the jury is out on whether being overweight has a negative effect on male fertility, being obese is a different story. There is increasing evidence that being obese may negatively affect sperm, due in part to increased inflammation, altered sex hormone production and damage caused to the DNA in sperm, known as 'sperm DNA fragmentation'.[8] One study found that the more overweight a man is, the higher the risk of infertility, with an increased risk of 10% for every 9 kg above his healthy weight.[8] When the father is obese, there is also an increased risk of chronic disease in his children,[5] so it is vital, not just for the health of the father but also for the health of his future children and grandchildren, that measures are put in place to reduce body weight. Support is vital for this to happen as excess weight is never just because someone eats too much and moves too little. There are always so many factors and a sympathetic GP/doctor as the initial point of contact has the potential to make a huge difference.

Being underweight can also impact fertility. This means having a BMI below 18.5, which can increase the risk of an abnormal menstrual cycle, with irregular or absent periods, making trying to conceive more of a challenge. With reduced food intake and potentially a less diverse diet, there is also the risk of nutritional deficiencies which can not only impact the woman's health but also that of her unborn child should she fall pregnant. There is also an increased risk of preterm delivery and low birth weight.[9] In the study where the BMI range for male fertility was larger than for women, the authors also found that being underweight significantly affected the chance of pregnancy. If both partners were underweight there was a 10% reduced chance of pregnancy, the same as if both were obese.

So, even though studies suggest that it is primarily a woman's fertility that appears to decline with any increase in BMI above the healthy range, and that men's fertility only appears to be affected in obesity, it is still sensible for both men and women to try and achieve a healthy weight prior to trying to conceive, both for their own health and for that of their future child. Current guidelines for weight management support are only written with women in mind and this may prevent men from seeking help. This really should not be the case as supported weight loss can help to improve male fertility as well as female, so please do ask for help if you are male and feel it will benefit your fertility journey.

Studies have shown that if men classed as obese lose weight sensibly, in other words avoiding rapid weight loss in the form of a crash diet, semen parameters can be improved. One study looked at obese men, with some being morbidly obese (BMI between 33 and 61) who took part in a 14-week diet and exercise programme and lost approximately 4-24% of their body weight.[10] A higher BMI range was associated with lower sperm concentration and count, lower motility and abnormal structure, and the men in the highest BMI range had a 71% lower sperm concentration, and a 68% lower total sperm count than the group with the lowest BMI, although they were still classed as obese. When looking at the weight loss, the group with the highest weight loss had a significant increase in total sperm count and in the size/shape of the sperm. In terms of hormones, obesity was associated with a reduction in testosterone, but those men who managed the greater weight loss had increases in testosterone and better overall hormone balance. It is important to highlight that, although there were improvements in hormone levels, they did not return to normal, healthy levels. This reflects the fact that the participants remained in the obese category despite the weight loss and highlights the importance of trying to achieve a healthy weight prior to trying for a baby.

Although BMI is often used as a sole measurement in determining whether someone is a healthy weight, it does have its limitations and I always prefer to use additional measurements in my assessments. These include measuring waist circumference, as this gives a better overall picture.

This measures the fat around your middle that builds up around your organs and is linked to an increased risk of chronic disease including heart disease and type 2 diabetes. To measure your waist circumference place a tape measure around your waist at the halfway point between the bottom of your ribs and the top of your hips. Make sure the tape measure is snug but not tight and breathe normally.

Reference range for people of White European, Black African, Middle Eastern and Mixed origin

	Men:	Women:
Low risk	Below 94 cm	Below 80 cm
High risk	94-102 cm	80-88 cm
Very high risk	More than 102 cm	More than 88 cm

Reference range for people of African Caribbean, South Asian, Chinese and Japanese origin

	Men:	Women:
Low risk	Below 90 cm	Below 80 cm
Very high risk	Above 90 cm	Above 80 cm

(NB There is no 'high risk' category for this second group)

8

Oxidative stress

How does oxidative stress affect fertility?

Oxidative stress is quite a complicated process so I will try and break it down for you as it took me a long time to get to grips with it in university! When we breathe in oxygen our cells use the vast majority of it for energy generation, but a very small percentage is wasted and the oxygen splits into single atoms (the chemical formula for oxygen is O_2, meaning it contains two oxygen atoms). These single atoms are called 'free radicals' and they are very unstable and reactive; they stumble around bumping into other molecules and reacting with them, much like someone who has had too much alcohol at a party and crashes around, bumping into people and becoming aggressive. This reaction is called oxidation and this actually is an everyday occurrence in our bodies and to some degree we need this to happen in order to function properly. For example, if we have an infection, we need these molecules to help fight off the bugs and enable us to recover. For fertilisation to occur we also need a small number of free radicals. The problem occurs when too many are produced.

The way our bodies maintain harmony is to have an even number of these free radicals and antioxidants which our bodies produce but which are also provided by the food we eat. This is because the antioxidants' job is to stabilise the free radicals and prevent them from causing damage to our cells and DNA. It is when there is an imbalance that things get tricky as without the actions of the antioxidants, the free radicals are at liberty to rampage and it is at this point they begin to cause damage: known as 'oxidative stress'.

It is not just the processes within our bodies that cause oxidative stress though. There are many external factors and these include certain components of animal foods, low intakes of whole foods, stress, smoking, environmental pollutants, heavy metals and alcohol.

As well as being associated with an increased risk of many health conditions, oxidative stress is associated with poor fertilisation, miscarriage, birth defects and poor embryo development. Women with endometriosis have been found to have high levels of oxidative stress in the cells that surround the developing egg which may result in poorer quality oocytes (immature eggs).[1] It has also been recognised as a probable cause of unexplained male infertility due to damage to the sperm. Sperm in particular are very easily damaged once they are formed, and studies have shown that men with higher levels of oxidative stress are less fertile than men with lower levels.[2] Studies have also shown that oxidative stress in semen is associated with poorer fertility treatment outcomes, including lower fertilisation rates, failed embryo development and implantation, recurrent miscarriage and lower live births.[3]

The maturing egg can also be damaged, and for these reasons it is important to minimise exposure to all the things we can control that result in oxidative stress. This means eating nutrient-dense foods, including those with antioxidant properties, and improving our lifestyles so that we can optimise not just the health of our sperm and eggs but our general health too.

Over the following chapters, we will look at the impact of nutrition, sleep, stress, exercise, environmental toxins, alcohol and caffeine on fertility, and also discuss the importance of supporting each other, if this is applicable, through each other's fertility journey. I want to start though with how diets high in animal products can impact fertility.

9

Animal foods and effects on fertility

As the title of this book implies, I recommend a plant-based diet to optimise fertility in both men and women. Ideally that translates into a whole food approach where all animal products are eliminated. This is based on both my personal and professional experience, and on the research I have read. However, I am also aware that many of you may not be ready to adopt this dietary pattern but would still like to make some positive changes that will help to optimise your fertility. If you are nodding your head at this I would strongly recommend you start by reducing animal products, with the emphasis being on meat; you will read the reasons for this shortly. When I speak to my patients about reducing, or eliminating, the animal products in their diet, I like to explain the evidence-base behind why this is beneficial as men in particular can often be reluctant to change their eating habits, especially if their diet is meat heavy.

Animal protein

We have data from a large study called the Nurses Health Study II (this study has been ongoing since 1991), which looked at over 18,000 women without a history of infertility as they attempted to become pregnant over an eight-year period. The data showed that higher intakes of animal protein were associated with higher rates of ovulatory infertility, with chicken and turkey surprisingly having more of an effect than red meat.[1] Having just one extra daily portion of animal protein, but in particular poultry and red meat, significantly increased the risk of ovulatory infertility, but replacing this with plant protein resulted in a significantly reduced risk. The authors explained one reason might be the beneficial effects of plant protein in lowering insulin resistance, but the presence of the amino acid, arginine, may also have something to do with it. Arginine is involved in the making of nitric oxide in the body and this is really important for good blood flow to the male and female reproductive organs, as discussed in Chapter 2.

One type of fertility treatment option is intracytoplasmic sperm injection (ICSI), and this is the most common treatment when the cause of infertility is sperm-related. It is different to IVF as instead of leaving the sperm and egg to fertilise by themselves, a sperm is injected directly into the egg. For women going through this type of treatment it has been shown that those who eat more red meat have a reduced chance of blastocyst development.[2] A blastocyst is a ball of cells made by the egg around four to five days after it has been fertilised by the sperm and is the early stage of embryo development. Blastocyst formation was shown to be positively associated with fish intake; however, this does not necessarily mean it is the fish itself that is giving the benefits. It is much more likely to be the nutrients contained in fish and, as you will read shortly, it is possible to consume all of these nutrients via plant-based sources if you choose not to eat fish.

Meat is also a vector for exposure to hormones and antibiotics (with the exception of organic versions, though this does not mean these are better for fertility as I will discuss) and there is the very real possibility that antibiotic resistance could affect fertility in both men and women. This is because the infections that are becoming increasingly resistant include sexually transmitted infections, and if these are left untreated they can lead to permanent damage to reproductive function. Healthy animals in some countries are given antibiotics as a growth promoter to increase profits, and although the US and Europe have banned this practice, they still allow prophylactic use. This means the animals are given antibiotics to prevent disease as well as treating it, with the dose being higher than that used for growth promotion.[3]

In some countries, around 80% of antibiotic use is in animals and, as we are exposed to these medicines by eating them, it is contributing to the rising threat of antibiotic resistance. This means that common illnesses and infections that have been successfully treated with antibiotics in the past are now becoming increasingly more difficult to treat as the bacteria are resisting the effects of the medication. A shocking report was published in the *Lancet* recently. This reported the global estimates for deaths associated with resistance to antibiotics used to treat bugs that cause infection in our bodies. It was estimated that in 2019 over 1.2 million people died directly as a result of this, with one of the top two bugs most likely to cause death being *E. coli*, a common species. Worryingly, it has been estimated that antibiotic use will have increased by 67% by 2030, with some countries using significantly more.[3] The World Health Organization (WHO) has set guidelines strongly recommending an overall reduction in antibiotic use in food-producing animals, with complete restriction for growth promotion and use in healthy animals.

What else in animal products can harm our fertility?

Advanced glycation end products (AGEs)

There are other components in meat, dairy and eggs that have been associated with poorer fertility outcomes. As well as saturated and trans fats (see page 121), these include advanced glycation end products, or AGEs. I don't want to get too deeply into the science around AGEs but they are basically formed in the body when sugars attach to proteins. There are many routes for the entry of AGEs into our bodies: they are made internally but there are also outside sources, including our diet, alcohol and smoking. They are a known risk factor for heart disease and stroke as they can stiffen our arteries, but they are also associated with decreased male and female fertility.

We have receptors throughout our body for AGEs, including throughout the male and female reproductive tract. When they attach to these receptors they can cause damage to cells and DNA, and cause inflammation. In men, they may cause damage to the DNA in sperm, and reduce sperm quality,[4] and in women they can accumulate around the ovaries and inside the uterus. This can lead to early ovarian aging and failure of the embryo to implant. Women with polycystic ovary syndrome (PCOS) have been shown to have more than twice the circulating levels of AGEs and this in part is due to AGEs increasing insulin resistance. Our bodies produce insulin, a hormone, to allow our fat and muscle cells to take up glucose from our bloodstream. It also allows our livers to store it. In insulin resistance, the hormone is less effective and we have to produce more and more insulin from the pancreas to encourage our cells to take glucose up. Initially this isn't a problem, but over time if it continues to happen the cells in the pancreas that produce the insulin can wear out and they cannot produce enough insulin to overcome the resistance. This then results in high blood glucose levels and ultimately the development of type 2 diabetes.

Reducing dietary AGEs is a really important part of dietary recommendations for all women and men trying to conceive, but particularly for women with PCOS which is the most common cause of infertility in women of reproductive age (see Chapter 4).

Cigarettes are one of the highest sources of AGEs but if you are trying to conceive, you are hopefully not smoking. So where else do these AGEs come from and how can we reduce them? Well, the highest dietary sources are cooked meat and animal products, as although they are naturally present in raw animal products, when they are heated, especially if they are cooked with a dry heat, new

AGEs are formed. This includes frying, barbequing, baking, roasting and grilling. If you are considering reducing the animal products in your diet, meat is the best place to start. Some people find it easy to reduce or even eliminate meat overnight but for others it may take months or even years to make sustainable, long-term adjustments to their diet. If that is the case for you, especially if you have a partner who is not willing to give up meat, what steps can you take in the meantime to reduce exposure?

Ways to reduce AGE exposure

Changing your cooking method can immediately start to reduce, but not eliminate, the AGEs you consume and you can do this by adding moisture and preventing the brown layer from forming on the meat you cook. Preferable cooking methods would be poaching, casseroling, steaming and slow cooking. You can also change the acidity of foods – for example, marinading meat in lemon juice and/or vinegar will reduce the AGE formation when cooked. Clinical trials have shown that such strategies for reducing the AGE formation in food is associated with up to a 50% reduction in AGE content of the diet. You can still significantly reduce your exposure by changing your cooking methods and reducing your overall meat intake, so if your partner continues to eat meat, or if you struggle to eliminate it entirely yourself, these strategies will be beneficial.

When you are starting to reduce your meat intake, it is important to replace those foods with plant-based protein alternatives. There are so many to choose from, including tofu, tempeh, edamame beans, lentils, chickpeas, beans and whole grains. It is important to be aware that there are ways that AGEs can be increased in plant foods – for example, roasting cashews more than trebles their AGE content compared to their raw state – so I would always advise you to eat unroasted, unsalted nuts to gain the most nutritional benefits.

Highly processed foods, and sugar-sweetened foods and drinks, are also rich sources of AGEs and should be minimised or avoided, not just for this reason but for the other components found in such products. I would say the most important thing to try and exclude from your diet altogether is sugar-sweetened drinks. These have been shown to increase the risk of obesity and other disease states, including type 2 diabetes and heart disease, and can often contain seriously high amounts of added sugar. For example, one can of cola contains around nine teaspoons of sugar! Swapping to diet versions to avoid the added sugar is not beneficial as they are full of artificial sweeteners and these too may be associated with reduced embryo quality and poorer outcomes for couples going through fertility treatment.[5]

What about dairy?

Dairy is a bit of a contentious topic as the data are conflicting. However, there is convincing evidence that high-fat dairy is associated with an increased risk of ovulatory infertility and this may be due to its saturated fat content.

In a paper discussing data from the Nurses Health Study II, no association was found between total dairy intake and the risk of ovulatory infertility, although low-fat dairy was associated with a higher risk and high-fat a lower risk.[6] This contradicts later studies which have shown higher saturated fat intakes to be counterproductive for fertility.

A recent review looked at a number of studies where dairy was examined in relation to its effects on fertility.[4] For women going through IVF, higher dairy intakes were associated with lower ovarian antral follicle counts. This is an ultrasound examination taken as part of fertility treatment to evaluate ovarian reserves. When there are fewer antral follicles developing on the ovaries (small fluid-filled sacs that each contain an egg), ovarian reserves are likely to be low, which means fewer eggs overall. There was also found to be an association between higher intakes of cream and yoghurt and a higher risk of irregular periods. Saturated fat was found to be associated with less mature oocytes being retrieved during IVF.

The review also found an association between men consuming higher dairy diets and lower total testosterone concentrations, as well as lower FSH and LH, all of which affect fertility.

There have been contradictory results from studies looking at dairy and fertility which means we can't draw definitive conclusions. However, there is convincing evidence that dairy is associated with poorer fertility parameters, especially in women going through fertility treatment. This may not be just because of its sometimes high saturated fat content but also due to its other components, including dietary AGEs, animal protein and small amounts of naturally occurring trans fats, all of which are associated with poorer fertility outcomes.

There are nutritional considerations of course. Dairy foods can be high in protein and calcium, and good sources of other nutrients, including vitamins D and B12, and iodine. It is therefore important to make sure that you take in enough of these nutrients if you are removing dairy from your diet. It is a common misconception, for example, that swapping dairy cheese for a plant-based cheese will mean a like-for-like swap when it comes to nutritional content, but actually most marketed vegan cheeses do not contain calcium and are very low in protein. They will also be high in saturated fat if they are made from coconut oil. A much better option is choosing nut or seed-based cheeses as these contain a wide range of micronutrients important for bone health and will be much lower in saturated fat. Some micronutrients found in dairy are not commonplace in a plant-based diet and these include vitamin D and iodine, although many would argue that as long as seaweed is eaten regularly this will provide all the iodine needed. I will discuss why this may not be a good idea in Chapter 13.

What about fish?

Fish is often associated with a healthy diet, particularly in terms of the Mediterranean diet where fish is eaten regularly. In the UK, NHS guidelines state we should eat at least two portions of fish a week, one of which should be an oily fish such as mackerel or salmon.

Why oily fish?

All fish contain omega-3 fatty acids, which you may have heard quite a lot about, but oily fish in particular contain much more. I won't delve too deeply into what omega-3s are here because I will be explaining in far more detail later on, but it is actually not the fish themselves that are the primary source of omega-3s. This is a common misconception fueled by the focus on oily fish as such rich sources. In fact, fish do not make their own omega-3; they accumulate them from the algae and plankton they eat, and also from the smaller fish on which they feed that have already accumulated omega-3 from the algae and plankton. It is not correct to say that without the inclusion of fish in the diet we will not be able to eat sufficient omega-3s, as we can simply cut out the middle man (aka the fish) and go straight to the source: the algae.

To do this in a way that is most effective, and to ensure that our bodies are absorbing efficiently, a vegan omega-3 capsule can be taken, and this must contain two important omega 3 fats: DHA and EPA (otherwise known as docosahexaenoic acid and eicosapentaenoic acid, those complicated names being the reason I only ever use the abbreviations!). There are no set dose guidelines, but based on the fact that eating one or two servings of fish per week (the Government recommendation for fish eaters mentioned above) gives you around 450 mg of EPA and DHA per day, I recommend 400-500 mg daily for both men and women trying to conceive who do not eat fish.

There is no denying that fish contain a range of beneficial nutrients. However, there are some important things of which to be aware. Pregnant women are advised not to exceed one portion of oily fish weekly due to the mercury content, with complete avoidance of higher mercury-containing fish such as swordfish and king mackerel. Fish and crustaceans have also been shown to contain pollutants and pesticides that are unfortunately ever increasing in our waters, and although these levels are unlikely to cause harm when eaten in the amounts humans consume, we do not know for sure what effects they may have on fertility and general health. Fish and seafood are also sources of microplastics and I will be discussing microplastics in more detail later (see Chapter 16). To give an example though: regular consumption of shellfish may expose you to over 11,000 microplastic particles a year,[7] a significant number. The reason for this is that shellfish filter seawater so take in any microplastics from that water. These microplastics can be found in concentrated amounts in the digestive tract of seafood, meaning that eating whole fish and seafood, such as whitebait and mussels, will expose you to higher numbers.

10

The power of plants

There are without question many highly beneficial effects of eating a predominantly whole food plant-based diet, but I want to make one thing very clear. A plant-based diet will not *guarantee* that you fall pregnant and carry to full term. Nothing can do that and anyone who claims otherwise is not only wrong but is giving false hope; I will not do that. What adopting a plant-based diet can do is help to *optimise* both male and female fertility to improve the chances of conceiving. It does this by creating an anti-inflammatory, antioxidant-packed environment, and positively impacting egg and sperm quality. Lifestyle changes alongside dietary changes also help to reduce stress, help you to sleep better, improve your fitness and help you to minimise or avoid substances that can negatively affect your fertility. All of these things combined can mean that a man is in the best health to provide his sperm, and a woman is in the best physical shape to prepare for and carry a baby.

A 'plant-based diet' can have several meanings. It can imply that you still include animal products but in lower quantities so that your diet is based around plant foods. It can also mean that you have eliminated all animal products and follow a diet based purely on plants. These are examples of a plant-based diet; you can see how varied the term can be:

- Lacto-vegetarian: Dairy foods are eaten, but eggs, meat, poultry and seafood are excluded
- Ovo-vegetarian: Eggs are included but all other animal foods are avoided

- Lacto-ovo-vegetarian: Dairy and eggs are eaten, but meat, poultry and seafood are excluded
- Flexitarian: Animal products are occasionally eaten
- Pescatarian: Fish and shellfish are eaten, but all other animal products are avoided
- Vegan: All animal products are excluded
- Whole food plant-based: All animal products are excluded and the majority of food eaten is in its whole form, so focusing on whole grains, legumes, nuts, seeds, fruit and vegetables.

The majority of studies where plant-based diets have been examined have looked at plant-predominant diets, meaning that small amounts of animal products are still consumed. The most studied diet in these terms is the Mediterranean diet, where the emphasis is on a variety of fruit and vegetables, beans, whole grains, nuts, seeds, olive oil and fish, with lower amounts of meat and dairy. It would be wrong to say the evidence is clear that following a whole food plant-based diet will give greater benefits in terms of fertility compared to following a plant-predominant diet. This is important for those trying to conceive who are wanting to make big improvements to their diet but do not necessarily want to remove every animal product. Any positive change will give some degree of benefit and if that means still including some non-processed meat, fish, eggs or dairy but building the majority of meals around plants, that is okay. The most important thing is that eating does not become a stressful event as this is counterproductive in itself.

My belief though, and this is based on the growing evidence-base, is that following a predominantly whole food plant-based diet really will deliver the most benefits, not just in terms of fertility but also for overall physical and mental health. I also believe that a diet pattern shouldn't be regimented, so the inclusion of some foods considered to be less healthy is absolutely okay. This could be a plant-based burger when eating out, or vegan ice cream when watching a film with friends, or a pizza on a Friday night. It is really important though to get the right support initially if you are thinking of switching to a plant-based way of eating. This will help to ensure that, if animal products are removed, your diet remains nutritionally complete. There are an awful lot of nutrition myths out there (some of which I debunk later), peddled by those without in-depth knowledge of nutritional science, so I would strongly urge you to only seek support from a registered dietitian or registered nutritionist, preferably one specialised in plant-based nutrition.

Many patients who come to see me are either already plant-based or are strongly considering it but are worried about how they will manage without certain foods. The key one tends to be dairy. I totally get it because that was the one thing I thought I would really struggle with, but there are so many brilliant dairy substitutes available, including the most amazing variety of chocolate! I can honestly say that I haven't missed it, at all. The key point is to ensure they you are still getting enough of the micronutrients contained in dairy, especially calcium because some dairy substitutes don't contain any at all. It is vital that you meet your daily calcium needs during pregnancy and lactation, and at every other time in your life in order to optimise your bone health, and I will explain how to do this in Chapter 13.

I love to watch my patients begin to reduce the animal products in their diet, and replace them with plants, because they start to feel so much better generally that most decide going fully plant-based is the next logical step. Some do struggle to eliminate animal products, and this may be for many different reasons. Maybe certain foods emotionally connect them to their childhood, or they can't imagine how their favourite meal can be replicated using plant foods. This is so common but it is actually a really fun challenge for me. There is nothing I love more than helping them to 'veganise' their favourite meal and show them how easy and how tasty plant-based cooking can be. Of course, some will decide that even though they really enjoy plant-based meals and have reduced the amount of animal products they eat, they are not ready to go fully plant-based, and again this is totally okay. Everyone is different and as long as you try to base meals around plants you will naturally be increasing your intake of fibre and fertility-friendly micronutrients and plant compounds. You will also be reducing your intake of saturated fat, haem iron (the iron found in animal products, more on that later – see page 164) and other components that can be less beneficial to fertility.

So, what does the ideal plate look like? My advice is to think about your main meals in terms of percentages (see Figure 8). So, fill 45% with a variety of vegetables, 5% with a great source of unsaturated fat, 25% with minimally processed protein and 25% with starchy carbohydrate-containing foods, preferably whole grains although if you opt for more refined carbohydrates every now and then that is fine too. When I say starchy carbohydrates I mean things like pasta, rice, potatoes, grains like couscous, bulgar wheat or 'pseudograins' like quinoa, amaranth and buckwheat. This label separates them slightly from whole grains because technically they are a seed but they have a very similar nutrient profile to whole grains and are eaten in the same way.

Is a vegan diet always a healthier choice?

It is a common belief that a vegan diet is automatically a healthier choice than a standard Western diet, but actually this isn't necessarily the case, and it is where the terms 'whole food plant-based' and 'vegan' can have different meanings in the health context. Whereas the former focuses on eating foods mainly in their whole form, so focusing on whole grains, nuts, seeds, legumes, fruit and vegetables, a vegan diet can often mean relying on more heavily processed

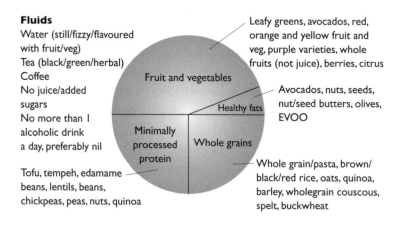

Fluids
Water (still/fizzy/flavoured with fruit/veg)
Tea (black/green/herbal)
Coffee
No juice/added sugars
No more than 1 alcoholic drink a day, preferably nil

Tofu, tempeh, edamame beans, lentils, beans, chickpeas, peas, nuts, quinoa

Leafy greens, avocados, red, orange and yellow fruit and veg, purple varieties, whole fruits (not juice), berries, citrus

Avocados, nuts, seeds, nut/seed butters, olives, EVOO

Whole grain/pasta, brown/black/red rice, oats, quinoa, barley, wholegrain couscous, spelt, buckwheat

Fruit and vegetables

Healthy fats

Minimally processed protein

Whole grains

Figure 8: The ideal plate

foods, and a diet high in these types of food means a diet high in saturated fat, sugar, salt and other less healthful components.

You just have to go into the supermarkets and look at the expanding plant-based aisles to see the quantity of ultra-processed foods that are appearing on the shelves. From crispy tofu bites, to quiches, to pizzas, meat substitutes and pies, the choice is huge. While such foods are certainly preferable to processed animal products, they can still be high in ingredients that can negatively affect egg and sperm quality, the health of the lining of the womb and the implantation process. They are also much lower in fibre than whole foods because the food in these products has been so broken down that much of the nutrient profile has been stripped away. As some of the ingredients act as stressors to our bodies, more antioxidant-containing foods also need to be eaten to try and counteract the damage, and that won't be happening if you are not eating enough whole foods.

I'm not saying that you need to avoid all ultra-processed vegan foods to optimise your fertility because, in small amounts, I do believe certain options have their place. For example, one of the pillars of lifestyle medicine is the nurturing of healthy relationships and one of the most enjoyable ways to spend time with loved ones is catching up over a meal out, either in a restaurant or at someone's house. During these social occasions, it may not be possible to have a whole food meal, especially if someone else is doing the cooking or you are in a non-vegan restaurant, so having a plant-based burger or pizza may be the only option. The key is finding the right balance and I always stand by the 80/20 rule: eat a diet packed with whole foods 80% of the time, and enjoy non-whole foods 20% of the time. This allows for flexibility and a healthy relationship with food.

It can be difficult to swap processed foods with whole foods because your taste buds will be used to the flavours of processed food. The fact they can be high in saturated fat, sugar and salt means that they can have a nice mouth feel and can taste more flavoursome than foods which are naturally low in all of these things. They can also be addictive as they immediately light up the pleasure centre in the brain, so the more you have the more you want. The good news is though, you can retrain your tastebuds to take pleasure from foods low in salt, sugar and saturated fat and it can take as little as a week.

Once you start experimenting with whole foods, you will be amazed at how much flavour you can pack into your meals by just adding some spices and herbs, and/or a squeeze of fresh lemon or lime. You will really start to appreciate the beautiful, natural flavours of fruit and vegetables, and marvel at how much choice is out there. Be patient though because you may not like the first meal you make if you are new to the whole food approach, especially if you are swapping a pizza for a chickpea curry with brown rice, or cooking with tofu for the first time (trust me when I say that my first tofu meal was the most tasteless meal I have ever cooked and my husband would be more than happy to testify to this!). I promise you though, once you have mastered the herbs, spices and marinades, and your tastebuds have acclimatised, you will absolutely love it.

It's funny because so many people have said to me 'but don't you find your diet restrictive and boring?', when actually nothing can be further from the truth. I would argue that the standard Western diet is restrictive and boring. I know when I ate animal products, my meals would be very repetitive, consisting of a piece of meat or fish, a couple of vegetables, and either potatoes, rice or pasta. Now, I eat a variety of grains, including many I didn't even know existed, like freekeh and black rice. I eat a whole rainbow of fruit and vegetables, experiment with all the different ways you can cook tofu, and I love finding independent vegan restaurants near me to try out. By the way, if you live in Cardiff or are planning to visit, Luna's Vegan Corner on Wellfield Road is a must. Their tofu buddha bowl is the best you will ever have and there is always enough left over for lunch the next day, no matter how hungry you are when you start eating it.

What about oils?

The topic of oils splits the plant-based community in two, with some strongly advocating for no oils and others being happy to include them. I fall into the latter category and the main message I want to give here is that not all are equal.

There are two main plant-based oils that contain high levels of saturated fat and for this reason I would advise minimising or avoiding them completely as high levels of saturated fat in the diet increase the risk of heart disease, and also negatively affect fertility. These are coconut oil and palm oil, and despite many people claiming coconut oil has health benefits, it does not. The saturated fat content is equal to lard and you certainly wouldn't want to include that in your diet on a regular basis. Palm oil is also very high in saturated fat and is also damaging in terms of its environmental impact, even if it claims to be sustainably sourced.

Predominantly unsaturated fats like vegetable oil and olive oil can be included as part of a healthy diet. Extra virgin olive oil (EVOO) in the modest quantities you would tend to use in cooking, is associated with lower rates of cardiovascular disease, and as this can be an underlying cause of sexual dysfunction in men and women it can be a positive inclusion in the diet. If you are trying to watch your overall energy intake, then certainly reducing the amount of oil you are using will be beneficial but you do not need to cut it out completely if you do not want to. There are ways in which you can cook without oil – for example, using a little water or stock to saute onions and garlic – and for some this works well but it is a personal preference so just choose whatever works for you, and remember that we need a certain level of fat to produce hormones and absorb fat-soluble vitamins, both of which are essential for healthy reproductive function.

11

Phytonutrients

What are phytonutrients and how can they help fertility?

The word 'phytonutrient' (interchangeably used with phytochemical) comes from the Greek word phyton, meaning plant, and refers to the compounds in or derived from plants that have health benefits both to the plant itself and to humans.

Phytonutrients may counteract the actions of free radicals by exerting antioxidant, anti-inflammatory and anti-antimicrobial actions, and have positive effects on cardiovascular health and immune functions. Their antioxidant, anti-inflammatory actions in particular mean they are essential compounds to include in the diet to help protect sperm and egg quality. As they also help to reduce inflammation in the body, they promote a more optimal internal environment for conception. The basic rule is to 'eat the rainbow', a term commonly referred to in the plant-based community. What this means is that, by including as many different coloured fruit and vegetables in your diet as you can, you will be consuming a wide range of phytonutrients, all of which have slightly different or mutual benefits on the body. By eating in-season varieties, you will be eating even more concentrated quantities of these compounds because they are much fresher and have higher nutritional value.

The most common types of phytonutrient are polyphenols (over 8000 different polyphenols have been found in the food we eat) which make up over 60% of all phytonutrients,[1] and include anthocyanins, flavanols, flavonols, phenolic acids, stilbenes, isoflavones and flavanones, among others.

Anthocyanins

Anthocyanins are found in high concentrations in the foods we eat and are derived from red, violet and blue flowers and their fruit. More than 600 have been identified and the richest food sources include black elderberries, blackcurrants and blueberries. An interesting fact about blueberries is that, although the larger ones may seem more appealing and are often sweeter, the smaller more bitter berries contain more anthocyanins and are a better choice if you really want to pack an antioxidant punch. You will also find them in red berries and apples, cherries and coloured vegetables, including red onions, aubergines and red lettuce.

I often hear it said that wine contains polyphenols and for this reason it is 'good for you'. I go into alcohol in more detail in Chapter 16, but looking specifically at polyphenol content, let's compare for example red wine and black tea. Both have comparable amounts of polyphenols but the big difference lies in their effects on the body. Wine contains alcohol which acts as a source of oxidative stress, whereas tea does not contain alcohol, meaning all the antioxidant activity of the polyphenols it contains can exert their positive effects on the body without the alcohol counteracting some of those effects. If your main concern is getting more polyphenols into your diet, I would focus on achieving your aim by eating a range of plant foods rather than including red wine as a useful source.

Flavanols

Flavanols can also be found in a wide range of foods, including cocoa and dark chocolate, nuts, coffee and black tea.

Flavonols

Flavonols can be found in fruit, vegetables and tea, with quercetin being one of the most commonly known types of flavonol. It is found in high quantities in onions, cranberries and berries.

Phenolic acids

Phenolic acids are present in herbs and spices, as well as in fruit such as wild blueberries and plums, vegetables such as aubergines and carrots, cocoa, tea and coffee.

Stilbenes and flavanones

You will probably recognise stilbenes more as resveratrol, which is found in grapes, wine and citrus fruit. There are resveratrol supplements on the market but they are pricey and can be as high a dose as 350 mg per capsule which is significantly higher than any dose you would get from food. This may have potentially damaging rather than beneficial effects as more is not always better. As is usually the case, eating whole foods enables you to get what you need without risking excess.

Isoflavones

The only source of these polyphenols in the diet are soya beans, so you will benefit from any soya product, including tofu, tempeh and edamame beans. You will also find lesser amounts in soya milk and yoghurts as these are more processed but are still useful additions to the diet, especially for the micronutrients contained in the fortified versions.

The importance of variety

How many of these food sources do you eat on a weekly basis? If you find, like a lot of people, you've fallen into the trap of eating the same types of plant food regularly, now is a good idea to switch it up. One way you can do this is by tearing up the shopping list which you probably write on autopilot (I know I often do) and go to the supermarket with an open mind. Take time browsing the fresh produce aisles and put a few things in your trolley that you do not usually eat and have no idea what to do with. You can also do this with frozen fruit and vegetables. You will be amazed just how much variety is out there that you have not noticed before and if you have to look up how to cook something you will discover new recipes and new flavours at the same time.

When it comes to how many phytonutrients we should be eating per day, there are no guidelines for this and I wouldn't get too fixated on aiming for a set amount. As long as your goal is a minimum of 30 different plant foods a week, you will be getting all you need. A good way of initially checking your intake is to make yourself a card with the different food groups on it and then place a mark in each box every time you eat a food from that group. Remember that eating three apples will only count as one mark as the aim is to eat as wide a variety as you can, and herbs and spices only count as ¼ of a plant point each, so to get one point you will need to have four different herbs and spices. Figure 9 shows what your card could look like.

Fruit	||||	Vegetables	||||
Whole grains	卌	Nuts	|||
Seeds	|||	Legumes	||||
Herbs	||||	Spices	|||

Figure 9: A sample food group chart showing an ideal balance

In time you won't need to use a card like this as your diet will be packed with plant foods, but it can be a really useful way of keeping on track when you are first starting out.

12

The gut microbiota

We know that to have the best chances of conceiving we need to be in good physical and mental health and neither of these things is fully possible without a well functioning internal environment of micro-organisms. This sounds strange doesn't it? Surely bacteria are harmful – things that cause illness and disease? This is certainly true for some bacteria, but actually the bacteria in your gut can be the key to improved immunity, and a lower risk of a number of conditions, including depression, anxiety and even Alzheimer's disease.

We have around 100 trillion micro-organisms, including bacteria, fungi and viruses, colonising every area of our body, including on our skin and in the cavities in our bodies.[1] We are basically a seething mass of all of these things which sounds pretty gross when you think about it! Collectively these organisms are called microbiota, making up the microbiome, and the highest concentration of these live in our gastrointestinal tract, especially in our colon (large intestine). Interestingly, by the age of 5 years, our gut microbiota are pretty much set to what they will be as an adult, and once established, the composition remains the same throughout our adult lives. However, there are many factors that can alter the composition, including excess weight, stress, antibiotic use, bacterial infections, smoking, disease states, medical treatment, surgical procedures and long-term dietary habits.[1]

The bacteria in our gut (there can be over a thousand different types inside us) help us to break down the food we eat, and that means releasing the nutrients and components of that food. Our bacteria are like us; they need food to survive and grow, and like us they also need the right type of food. It is important we feed our bacteria as diverse a range of fibre-containing foods as possible so we can also have a diverse range of bacteria. Low bacterial diversity is associated with a wide range of conditions, including obesity, autoimmune diseases such as inflammatory bowel disease and rheumatoid arthritis, and neurological conditions such as dementia and Alzheimer's disease. It has also been associated with poorer response to vaccinations.[1]

When our gut bacteria are less diverse, this results in what is called dysbiosis (basically an imbalance) and this allows opportunistic inflammatory bacteria to grow that can crowd out the anti-inflammatory bacteria. This can have a significant effect on the gut because, when there is harmony, the anti-inflammatory bacteria protect the wall of the colon, keeping it strong. However, when there is dysbiosis, this protection decreases and the wall can get damaged, meaning an increase in intestinal permeability (the medical term), or 'leaky gut' as it is often called. This can result in widespread inflammation and an increased risk of many diseases, including cardiovascular disease, type 2 diabetes, autoimmune conditions and many others. The inflammation can also worsen symptoms of irritable bowel syndrome as the nerves and muscles of the gut lining can be affected. This means an increase in symptoms such as diarrhoea, constipation, abdominal pain and bloating, and it can also exacerbate symptoms of PCOS for women who experience gastrointestinal discomfort.

Often, people are given a diagnosis of 'leaky gut' by those who do not understand how the body works but actually this should never be a diagnosis on its own. Instead, it should be recognised that it is a sign something else is going on that should be investigated and addressed. From time to time we can all suffer from slightly increased intestinal permeability – for example, during times of stress, or after drinking too much alcohol at one time – but the gut typically recovers when these triggers are removed. However, if the triggers remain, the 'leaky gut' will continue. One example of this is someone with coeliac disease who continues to eat gluten because they have not yet seen a doctor for their gut symptoms and do not know the cause. This will trigger increased intestinal permeability and the only way to allow the gut to heal is to remove the gluten and follow a strict gluten-free diet. You can see then that there is an underlying cause in this situation: undiagnosed coeliac disease. This is something that urgently needs intervention to prevent the associated risks of continuing to eat foods that trigger the body's immune response. If someone with undiagnosed coeliac disease is given a diagnosis of 'leaky gut', it may mean their diagnosis by a medical doctor is delayed while they try and address ways in which to heal their gut. It is vital if you ever experience new gut symptoms, or have been having symptoms for a while but haven't been able to identify the cause, always to see your doctor as they will be able to investigate further and refer you to a specialist if needed.

Coeliac disease and fertility

Another important reason for my talking about coeliac disease here is that it can be an underlying cause of infertility if you do not know you have it and continue to eat gluten.

A common myth about coeliac disease is that it is an allergy or food intolerance. This isn't true; it is actually an autoimmune disease and, when someone with coeliac eats gluten, it causes damage to the lining of their small intestine. You cannot 'grow out of' being coeliac; it is a lifelong condition and a completely gluten-free diet, including the exclusion of wheat, barley and rye, is the only treatment.

Worryingly, Coeliac UK state that it takes on average 13 years to get a diagnosis, partly because the symptoms are so similar to IBS.

This is why over 60% of people living with coeliac in the UK are yet to be diagnosed.

If you have been struggling to conceive for some time and have been given a diagnosis of unexplained infertility, you should ask your GP to screen you for coeliac disease (this is in the NICE guidelines), which involves a simple blood test. It isn't clear why undiagnosed coeliac disease affects fertility, but one theory is that it is the result of the malabsorption that occurs when someone with coeliac continues to eat gluten. This malabsorption means that they can become deficient in a number of nutrients important for fertility, including zinc, iron, selenium and folic acid. Women with undiagnosed coeliac disease can also be underweight, which we know impacts fertility, and the fertile window may be shorter due to disruptions to hormones. The good news is there is no evidence that well managed coeliac disease affects fertility in men or women, so if you do have a positive diagnosis it is really important to see a specialist dietitian who will guide you through a gluten-free diet and other considerations.

Important information about testing for coeliac disease

If you awaiting a diagnosis and have identified foods, such as bread and pasta, as being triggers for your symptoms and have excluded them from your diet, it is really important to include at least one serving of gluten-containing food every day for six weeks before having your blood test. This means having a source of gluten every day in at least one meal, or having a daily sandwich with two slices of bread. The reason for this is that, when someone with coeliac eats gluten, the body releases antibodies in response and it is these antibodies that are detected in the blood test. If you remove gluten, the test will not detect these antibodies and you will get a false negative.

It doesn't end there though. If the blood test is positive, you will be sent for a more invasive test called a gastroscopy, where a camera is passed into your gut and a biopsy taken of the lining. You will also need to continue eating gluten for this test, the reason being that when someone with coeliac disease eats gluten, a reaction happens in the gut called villous atrophy. This is when the little finger-like projections in the lining of the small intestine, called villi, which help you to absorb nutrients from your food, flatten as a result of the damage caused. If gluten is removed, these villi repair and again you are likely to get a false negative result. I'm not going to pretend this process is pleasant, especially if you experience symptoms when eating gluten. However, it is really important to get a diagnosis if you do have coeliac disease, as then you can receive specialist help and in some cases find the underlying cause for your difficulties conceiving.

Returning to the gut microbiota then, how can we make improvements and prevent dysbiosis?

Ways to improve the gut microbiota

Well, the simple answer is to reduce the amount of animal protein and saturated fat in your diet and eat more plants as all plants contain that lovely, health promoting fibre. Fibre used to be separated into soluble and insoluble fibre but we are stepping away from that now as other qualities are thought to be more important. For example, the fibre (beta glucan) in foods such as oats and pulses forms a gel-like substance in the gut which can help reduce or delay the absorption of sugar and fats. Other types of fibre (called fermentable fibres) provide food for our gut bacteria. When we eat foods containing these fibres, such as beans, chickpeas, certain varieties of fruit and vegetables, and a variety of other plant foods they pass through our digestive system largely unchanged until they reach our colon. While our good bacteria start to break the food down and release all of the amazing nutrients it contains, something else really important happens; the bacteria also enable compounds called short chain fatty acids (SCFAs) to be released. The main three SCFAs are butyrate, acetate and propionate and these exert benefits on several organs, including the brain. If our diets are high in animal products and low in fibre, our anti-inflammatory bacteria do not have enough food and the more inflammatory bacteria start to thrive in their place. They do this by breaking down the other food eaten which provides less favourable nutrients, such as saturated fat and haem iron.

If a patient comes to me consuming a high-meat diet, my priority is to remove the red and processed meat. In the case of processed meat, this is because the World Health Organization (WHO) has classed it as a group 1 carcinogen since 2015.[2] This means there is convincing evidence that it causes cancer, and they have stated that for every 50 g of processed meat eaten a day, the risk of colorectal cancer is increased by 18%. That is really significant. In the case of red meat, it is classed as a 2a probable carcinogen, meaning that it may cause cancer, and there is a similar associated risk (17%) when eating 100 g of red meat daily. When you consider that a standard steak weighs around 225 g you can see how little 100 g really is. Animal meat consumption also reduces SCFA production, especially of butyrate. Plant protein on the other hand is associated with increased production of SCFs.[3]

Acetate, propionate and butyrate work together to exert their amazing benefits. Each plant food we eat, whether that be whole grains, nuts, seeds, fruit, vegetables or legumes, produces a different mix of SCFAs, and this is why a diverse plant-based diet is so important. SCFAs have a number of different roles – for example, they make the colon more acidic, which prevents the growth of inflammatory bacteria – and butyrate may also help to repair intestinal permeability, or 'leaky gut'.

We also know that our gut houses 70% of our immune system and that our brain and gut are in constant communication via the vagus nerve, the longest nerve in the body. It is known as the 'motorway' of the nervous system because it connects so many vital organs. It is also responsible for controlling the muscles used for swallowing. All of this means that a healthy, balanced gut environment may help to support both a healthy immune system and a healthy brain environment. On the opposite side, a poor gut environment may impact immune function and may also increase the risk of a number of brain disorders, such as depression, anxiety, insomnia, difficulties concentrating and memory problems. As the brain also communicates with the gut, stress can negatively impact gut function, and this then becomes a bit of a vicious cycle. It remains to be determined whether the changes in the gut microbiota are a result of brain dysfunction, or whether brain dysfunction is a result of changes in the microbiota, but stress management is still vital to gut health and I will discuss this in relation to fertility at length later in this book (see Chapter 15).

What about fermented foods?

Fermented foods, including tempeh, sauerkraut and kimchi, are excellent additions to the diet as they contain live microorganisms that may be beneficial to the gut and also to general health, lowering the risk of type 2 diabetes and cardiovascular disease. Fermented vegetables have also been associated with a reduced risk of asthma and dermatitis.[4]

As we know that creating a diverse range of microbial species in our gut promotes gut and general health, it makes sense that eating foods containing these micro-organisms will be beneficial. Some of these species will be destroyed upon entering our stomach acid, but many have the ability to survive digestion and reach our colons intact, ready to start exerting their benefits. However, it is thought that because they have not developed within the microbiota that live in our guts, they are treated as 'foreign' micro-organisms and for this reason they may not become permanent members of the microbiota community. This does not mean that they do not have their uses though as even if they are transient, they may still be able to influence the structure, function and diversity of the microbiota.[4] Interestingly, fermented foods may also be able to act as a vehicle for folate (vitamin B9) delivery to at risk populations. Although the fermented food may not contain folate itself, some strains of bacteria are actually able to produce it via their own metabolism. Therefore, specific strains known to produce folate could be combined in order to enhance production of this important vitamin, making fermented foods a useful source of folate both for women of child-bearing age and for pregnant mothers.

One fermented food, sourdough, can also benefit us nutritionally as, although the finished product does not contain live micro-organisms because the bacteria do not survive the baking process, the lactic acid bacteria in the starter may express enzymes responsible for breaking down phytates. Phytates are compounds with antioxidant capability and are found in whole grains, legumes, nuts and seeds, but they can bind to certain minerals, especially zinc, iron and manganese, which reduces their absorption in the body. If there are enzymes in sourdough that can break down phytates, it means we are able to absorb the minerals more effectively within the bread, especially if it is made using whole grain flour. This means including sourdough regularly in the diet can provide a useful source of fertility-friendly zinc and iron compared to other breads.

What about sweeteners?

Zero- or low-calorie sweeteners are often used to replace sugar when someone is trying to reduce their intakes. This can be beneficial in terms of total energy consumed over a day, to reduce the risk of tooth decay, or to help manage blood glucose levels. However, there is evidence that sweeteners can have a negative effect on the gut microbiota.[3] There are three that have been shown to disrupt the balance and diversity of the microbiota in humans: sucralose, aspartame and saccharin. If you are trying to cut down on the added sugar in your diet, I would advise weaning yourself off any sweetener altogether rather than replacing one with another. Your taste buds do adapt very quickly and there are many ways to sweeten dishes without the need for added sugars or sweeteners. Dates work really well, whether you chop them and add to your porridge, or blend them to use in bakes. The only caveat to this is, if you suffer with IBS, dates are likely to make your symptoms worse if you have too many. Very ripe bananas are also excellent, and, rather than adding maple syrup, try adding berries or other fruit instead. This also gives the added benefit of providing more fibre to drive a more diverse gut environment.

What about probiotic supplements?

Many people take commercial probiotics with the aim of improving their gut microbiota, especially following a course of antibiotics. However, there is little evidence that these are beneficial, and actually taking them after antibiotic treatment may in fact delay the repairing of the gut.[2] There is also the potential risk of introducing infection into those with compromised immune systems as probiotics are live bacteria. If a patient would like to trial probiotics, I support this but I do make it very clear that the evidence is limited and for this reason I am unable to recommend a specific strain of probiotic. My usual recommendations are to trial one brand for one month, and if you do not notice any improvements, you can either try a different brand or stop taking them.

Finally, there is growing evidence that changes in the microbiota during pregnancy, driven by things such as antibiotic use, stress and variations in diet, can influence the growing baby's microbiota, brain development and future behaviour. This demonstrates the importance of ensuring the gut environment of the mother isoptimal during the pre-conception period, in preparation for pregnancy. This can be achieved by significantly reducing/

eliminating the things that enable the inflammatory bacteria to grow and adding in the things that enable the anti-inflammatory bacteria to flourish. My top tips for ensuring a diverse and healthy gut environment are shown in the box.

How to ensure a diverse and healthy gut environment

- Aim to eat 30 or more different plant foods each week. These should include whole grains, nuts, seeds, legumes, fruit, vegetables, herbs and spices.
- Include fermented foods in your diet regularly; however, minimise miso as it is high in sodium and high levels of sodium are associated with an increased risk of stomach cancer.[5]
- Minimise consumption of artificial sweeteners and additives. Where you can, use fruit to sweeten, and try to drink water as your main drink. If you are used to drinking squash it can be a difficult transition but you will get there, I promise! I used to be a squash fiend but weaned myself off gradually and now find that when I do have it, it tastes really artificial – your taste buds really do adapt. There are also lots of ways to add more interest to a glass of water – try throwing in some mint leaves and lemon slices, or strawberry and cucumber slices. What you can also do in the summer months is freeze water with herbs and/or fruit in ice cube trays and then pop them in your glass.
- Minimise or eliminate animal proteins and replace them with plant proteins, including a range of legumes (especially soya), nuts and seeds.
- Practise stress management techniques (see Chapter 15).

13

Pillar 1: Nutrition

Food is essential to health. We need it to survive, but we also need it to maintain good brain function, to be able to tolerate exercise, sleep well, reduce the risk of catching colds and other viruses, heal well from injuries and infections... the list is endless. Unfortunately, many people do not fuel their body in the right way and this increases the risk of poor health as well as having a negative impact on fertility.

The idea of using food to optimise fertility appeared as far back as Hippocrates (he died around 370 BCE), where his writings described how men should be 'sober and well-nourished with appropriate foods'. Sadly, he advised women trying to conceive to eat boiled puppy and octopus, in addition to celery, cumin seeds and frankincense, but the idea of the importance of diet for fertility was already present all those years ago. It continued through the Middle Ages, when women were given stags' liver or blood to help them conceive, and men were advised to eat almonds with aniseed and salt to improve sperm quality.

The standard Western diet containing high levels of saturated fat, salt and sugar, and low levels of fibre, is not beneficial to fertility, gut heath or general health but is unfortunately the predominant diet followed by the UK population. Not only is such a diet a known risk factor for metabolic diseases like obesity, cardiovascular disease and diabetes, as well as dementia and cancer, among others, but it is also associated with poor sperm and egg quality. For women in particular the effects of lifestyle and nutritional factors on reproductive function have been demonstrated in studies looking at artificial reproductive technology (ART) outcomes. This is because, unlike in natural conception, every stage of the process can be evaluated rather than relying on estimated dates.

A recent, really interesting study looked at 752 couples undergoing ICSI treatment between 2015 and 2019 to assess the influence of maternal nutrition and lifestyle factors on reproductive outcomes.[1] The women were asked to complete a food frequency questionnaire before treatment started to see how frequently certain foods were eaten and it also included multiple choice questions on smoking and exercising habits. The food categories investigated were refined sugars, artificial sweeteners, soft drinks, alcoholic drinks, fruit, vegetables and legumes, milk and dairy, and white and red meat.

The results showed a significant negative association between smoking, alcohol, refined sugars and artificial sweeteners and the number of retrieved oocytes, as well as fertilisation rate and early embryo development rate. There were also significant negative effects on implantation, clinical pregnancy and live birth rates, and for smoking an increased risk of miscarriage. Positive associations for the quality and quantity of eggs retrieved, clinical pregnancy rate and implantation rate were found with vegetables and legumes. Exercising also had a positive association with egg quantity and clinical pregnancy rate.

Dose-dependent relationships were observed between smoking, alcohol, sugar and artificial sweeteners on implantation, alcohol on clinical pregnancy, and smoking and alcohol on live birth rate. This means the higher the intakes, the higher the risk of the adverse outcomes, so for example the more cigarettes smoked the bigger the impact on oocyte quantity. Exercising and consuming foods such as milk and other dairy products, legumes, vegetables and fish were associated with reduced rates of oocyte abnormalities. Exercising and eating legumes and vegetables were also associated with improved ovarian stimulation response and clinical pregnancy rates.

When we look at the positive outcomes associated with dairy and fish, it is important to ask what is it in those foods that led to the positive association. Is it the dairy and fish themselves or their components? As you will see shortly, there are a wide range of micronutrients essential for optimal sperm and egg health. These include certain B vitamins, vitamins A, D and E, zinc and selenium, as well as the macronutrients fat, carbohydrate and protein. Omega-3 fatty acids are also a really important component of the diet for fertility. Therefore, as dairy and fish contain many of these nutrients, this may have been a factor in the findings. The fact that legumes and vegetables were associated with positive outcomes gives strength to this as they also contain a range of nutrients known to be key for all aspects of maternal fertility, from egg quality through to implantation. These include iron, folate, zinc, vitamin C and, of course, fibre. Legumes are also a good source of protein and, as you may remember, substituting animal protein with plant protein is associated with higher fertility rates.

Unfortunately, the male partners were not included in this study as it would have been really interesting to see whether the same foods had the same effects on sperm as on the eggs. However, a small study focusing purely on vegan versus non-vegan males and sperm health shows promising results.[2] Twenty men (10 vegans, 10 non-vegans) were recruited for the study. They all had to abstain from sex and alcohol prior to sperm analysis, and were asked to keep their activity levels constant. All participants were non-smokers, did not drink alcohol and had a BMI within the healthy range. They also had to have no history of mumps due to the known risks to fertility, and be in general good health. Their samples were collected and routine analysis took place, as well as assessments for oxidative stress and sperm DNA damage.

The results showed that, although there were no significant differences between groups in relation to sample size, sperm viability or morphology, there were significant differences in total sperm count, total motility and DNA damage. The vegan men had significantly higher total sperm count and motility, whereas the non-vegan men had a higher percentage of sperm DNA damage.

Now this study was very small and we definitely need larger scale studies to follow up on these findings, but the results are still encouraging and provide further evidence that plant-based diets are associated with favourable effects on sperm parameters.

MACRONUTRIENTS

Macronutrients consist of carbohydrates, protein and fat, and it is the 'macro' part (meaning large) that gives us an idea of how important it is to include sufficient amounts in our diet. It is not necessary to 'count macros'; what is important is to ensure a good mix of all with each meal and not to be tempted to leave out good-quality carbohydrates because they are SO important.

Carbohydrates

Let me start by saying that carbohydrate-containing foods are vital, not just for fertility, but for overall health. Unfortunately, they are the foods often demonised (along with fats) and the trend for 'low carb' diets doesn't appear to be waning. When you are trying to optimise your fertility, restricting carbohydrates is one of the worst things you can do.

First of all, not all carbs are equal and it is important to differentiate between the various types. The key difference is between unrefined and refined carbohydrates, with the former being the most beneficial to health and fertility, and a big reason for that is the fibre content.

Unrefined carbohydrates

Unrefined carbohydrates are naturally found in whole foods and include fruit, vegetables, beans, nuts, seeds, whole grains such as brown rice, barley and wholemeal couscous, and pseudo grains such as quinoa and buckwheat. These foods are packed with all kinds of fertility-friendly micronutrients, but I'm going to focus on fibre here because it really does play a key role in optimising fertility, especially in hormone-driven conditions like PCOS and endometriosis. For women with PCOS, where good blood glucose control is essential, fibre helps prevent those spikes in insulin and blood glucose levels which can make the condition so much harder to manage.

Another important role fibre plays is to help maintain hormone balance and it does this in a specific way. Our livers are perfect detox organs (which is why we don't need to waste money or time on gimmicky detox diets), and they are continuously filtering out toxins and substances our bodies don't need, including excess hormones. If these hormones enter our intestines and we have plenty of fibre in there, they will bind with the fibre and be removed from our body in our poo. If we don't eat enough fibre, there will be nothing to bind with and they will re-enter our bloodstream and continue circulating.

Finally, fibre helps keep you full and satisfied after a meal. One reason is that beta glucan slows down the passage of foods such as oats, brown rice and mushrooms through your intestines which increases the amount of time it takes your body to digest that food. Another reason is the slow digestion of other types of fibre by your amazing gut bacteria, which is the reason these foods help to keep your blood glucose levels steady. This means that you are less likely to feel the need for fast energy-providing snacks in-between meals, which will benefit your health in the long term. Another way fibre helps keep you full is by the production of those SCFAs. These not only help to strengthen your immune system, improve your gut and brain health and reduce the risk of many chronic diseases, but they also help your brain to recognise that you are full. What better reasons to pack that fibre in?

A number of studies have found that aiming for 25-29 g of fibre daily is associated with better health outcomes,[3] and current recommendations are that we should be aiming to eat a minimum of 30 g daily. Unfortunately, as a nation we are not eating anywhere near that amount, with the average intake being around 18 g. That means that some people are eating a lot less. I would advise that you don't get too fixated on 30 g as to most people it doesn't really mean anything – how can you measure 30 g of fibre? All you need to do is aim for a source of whole grains with each meal as often as you can (remember the ideal plate on page 89). This means that, if you are eating out, or at a friend's house, or on holiday and the only option is white pasta, or white rice, or if you just feel like a bowl of mashed potato or white spaghetti one evening, that is perfectly okay. As long as the majority of the time you are trying to include whole grain sources in your meals, that is what counts. Also try to include plenty of vegetables, fruit and other great sources of fibre, such as lentils, chickpeas, beans, nuts and seeds, and soya foods like tofu and tempeh and edamame beans. That way you will be hitting the daily 30 g target easily, and probably exceeding it (see Table 3).

Important data on the benefits of whole grains comes from the EARTH (Environment and Reproductive Health) study, a large ongoing study looking at couples aged 18-46 undergoing fertility treatment at a clinic in the US. The data have shown that higher whole-grain intakes in the year before treatment started were associated with increased endometrial thickness on the day of embryo transfer and a higher probability of implantation and live birth, with implantation occurring in 70% of women with higher intakes of whole grains compared with 51% for women who had the lowest whole-grain intakes. These findings led the authors to conclude that an increase of one serving a day of whole grains was associated with a 33% increased chance of implantation and a 27% higher chance of a live birth.[5]

Table 3: Fibre content of some plant foods. (Source: Tesco online groceries and Pituch-Zadanowski et al, 2015[4])

Food	Portion size	Fibre content (g)
Apple	1 medium	3.7
Banana	1 medium	2.8
Kiwi	1 medium	2.6
Orange	1 medium	3.1
Mango	100 g	1.8
Broccoli	100 g	3
Carrots (cooked)	100 g	3.3
Cauliflower (cooked)	100 g	2.7
Sweetcorn	100 g	2.8
Chickpeas	120 g (half a can)	8.3
Beans	117 g (half a can)	9.4 (average)
Red lentils	80 g (cooked)	4.9
Multigrain bread	2 slices	3.5
Rye sourdough	1 slice	2.2
Oats	40 g	3.6
Weetabix	2 bix	3.8
Brown rice	75 g (uncooked)	4.3
Wholewheat pasta	75 g (uncooked)	6.8
Nuts	30 g	2 (average)
Chia seeds	30 g	10.2
Other seeds	30 g	4.4 (average)

The authors explained the beneficial effects of whole grains may be due to several factors, including the many antioxidant components that work together to prevent damage to the egg and sperm cells. Whole grains are also a source of lignans, the main source of phyto-oestrogens (see page 130) in a Western diet. These may act directly on endometrial tissue to increase thickness and the chance of implantation. Finally, the way in which fibre helps regulate insulin and blood glucose levels may contribute to whole grains' positive effects. If too much insulin is released as a result of insulin resistance so there are higher amounts in the blood than is normal, more androgens (e.g. testosterone) are released. At the same time, the proteins that stick to them to stop them circulating around the body, called sex hormone binding globulin or SHBH, are reduced. This means an excess of circulating androgens which can negatively affect the chances of implantation. On the other hand, when insulin production is reduced by diet – that is, eating higher-fiber foods – SHBG increases and androgen levels reduce, thereby creating a more welcoming womb environment.

Refined carbohydrates

Refined carbohydrates are the carbohydrates found in more processed grains, such as white flour, white rice and pasta, starches such as corn flour, and refined sweeteners such as white or brown sugar, or jam. Now I'm not going to demonise these foods as, again, they are not all equal. Refined grains still provide protein and a variety of micronutrients, but I would say try to eat these foods less often and focus more on unrefined carbohydrates, purely because they are higher in fibre and will have more beneficial effects on your gut health, hormone balance, blood glucose levels and fullness.

What we should be mindful of is the refined sweeteners, also known as added sugars. It is best to try to keep these to a minimum as they are associated with an increased risk of certain conditions such as type 2 diabetes, heart disease, obesity and tooth decay. World Health Organization (WHO) guidelines are that added sugars should make up no more than 5% of our overall daily energy requirements, and this is equivalent to 7 sugar cubes. This may sound like quite a lot but if you remember that one can of fizzy drink can contain 9 cubes, or even more, you can see that actually it is very easy to exceed this amount. It is also shocking to see just how much sugar is added to some foods. A well-known brand of bran flakes, for example, has sugar and glucose syrup added and provides just over 4 g of sugar per serving (30 g). When pouring your cereal from a large box, it is very easy to eat more than 30 g so potentially, in just your breakfast cereal, you could be eating over a teaspoon of added sugar.

Added sugars, as the name suggests, include sugar added to drinks and food. They also include the sugars in foods like honey, syrups and unsweetened fruit juices. Many cook books and social media accounts will claim that coconut sugar, date syrup, maple syrup and brown sugar are healthier alternatives to white table sugar, but this is not true. They are still all added sugars and will have the same effects on your blood glucose levels and dental health. Added sugars do not include sugars found naturally in fruit and vegetables, so please do not listen to anyone who tries to tell you that you should minimise fruit intake because fruit contains sugar. Yes, it does but it is not added sugar and, importantly, it comes packaged with a huge number of healthful nutrients and fibre.

If you are trying to cut down on added sugars, there are lots of ways to gradually reduce your intake. Try to replace where possible with fruit which is naturally sweet but comes packaged with lots of other important nutrients for fertility. Topping your breakfast with lots of fruit negates the need to add maple syrup or sugar, and there are many bake recipes where you can have fun experimenting with alternative sweeteners to sugar. I find for those where you have to use sugar, just reducing the amount in the recipe is an easy hack.

Most recipes work just as well with 75% of the sugar listed in the ingredients, and some work with dates, bananas and even apple sauce. I have had some absolute baking disasters using substitutes so don't expect it always to work, but you can have fun seeing what does work for you.

It really troubles me when I hear that women going through fertility treatment have been advised to go on a low-carb diet to improve their chances of conceiving, because it really is so damaging. Not only does it remove much of the fibre from your diet, but it also removes your body and brain's primary source of fuel. They love carbs! They need it for energy and the correct functioning of everything they do. Without carbs, you will quickly start to feel sluggish and fatigued, low in mood, and your concentration and memory will suffer. You will have less tolerance of exercise as your body will not be able to replenish its glycogen stores, and you can't use protein efficiently without carbohydrates, so your fitness gains will be reduced. This is because when you have insufficient carbohydrate-containing foods in your diet, your body will initially switch to using your fat stores for energy and will then use your protein stores. This means your muscles will be broken down rather than built up and any additional protein you eat will simply be used for energy.

Another big reason why cutting out carbs is not a good idea is that you will need to replace them with something to provide your body with all that lost energy and low-carb diets are often high in animal protein. As studies have shown, these are not fertility-optimising foods, quite the opposite, and aside from this, following a low-carb, animal-protein-heavy diet will result in other undesirable effects, including constipation and bad breath. In a nutshell, please never follow a low-carb diet if you are trying to conceive, and this goes for both of you if you have a partner. The very best thing you can do is ensure that your meals are balanced, with a great source of carbs, and choose snacks that contain both protein and carbohydrates. Examples would be nut butter with chopped banana, oat cakes with hummus, or a bowl of fruit with soya yoghurt and nuts and/or seeds sprinkled on top. Your reproductive system will thank you for it.

Carb-loving overnight oats

- 40 g rolled or jumbo oats if you like a chewier texture
- 2 tsp chia seeds
- 2 tsp pumpkin seeds
- 5 almonds
- 5 walnut halves
- ½ tsp ground cinnamon
- 100 ml plant milk (you may need more depending on preference)
- 2 tbsp Greek-style soya yoghurt
- Handful of frozen blueberries and raspberries

Method:
1. Put all the dry ingredients and fruit in a bowl, mix well, then top with the milk.
2. Pop in the fridge overnight then stir through the yoghurt in the morning and enjoy!

Fats

Like carbohydrates, not all fats are equal, and I see too many patients, women in particular, worry about eating any type of fat. Women need a certain amount of fat, especially when trying to conceive.

Fatty acids, which are the main components of fat, have so many roles in the body. They help us to absorb the fat-soluble vitamins A, D, E and K, all of which have positive effects on egg and sperm quality, and implantation. Fatty acids are needed to maintain the structure of our cells, and they are needed for good hormone health. They are also used as energy during the time a woman's egg is maturing and in early embryo development, so it is important that we get enough fat in our diets. The key is focusing on the right type of fat.

So, what are the different types of fat? Broadly speaking, they are divided into saturated and unsaturated fats, which occur naturally, and trans fats which mainly result from manufacturing processes.

Saturated fat

Saturated fatty acids are found in large amounts in animal products, and also in coconut and palm oil.

Unfortunately, among some groups, there exists the belief that saturated fat is not harmful and that eating a diet high in animal products can help improve fertility. At best this is not evidence-based, and at worst it is very likely to adversely affect your ability to conceive. A high intake of saturated fat is a known risk factor for cardiovascular disease, but this doesn't just increase your risk of suffering a heart attack or a stroke; it also increases the risk of sexual dysfunction. In men, this means erectile dysfunction, and in women lack of arousal, and lack of vaginal lubrication. Don't forget that your sexual organs are just that and they rely on good blood flow. If your arteries become clogged with plaque as a result of a highly saturated fat diet, this reduces the blood flow not just to your heart and lungs but to every organ in your body, including the penis and vagina.

A diet high in meat, dairy and eggs also often means that other more nutrient-rich, fertility-friendly foods are displaced and by that

I mean foods high in fibre and other beneficial nutrients and antioxidants. Saturated fats are not just found in animal products though; they can also be found in plenty of foods marketed for those following a vegan diet, again highlighting the difference between a whole food plant-based diet and a vegan diet pattern.

Trans fats

You have probably heard of the negative effects of eating trans fats and because of this it is commonly thought that they are a type of saturated fat. Actually, they are an unsaturated fat (as explained next) but this does not mean they are beneficial and should be included in the diet. When trans fats are made industrially to be added to many of the foods we eat, they are formed by adding hydrogen to vegetable oil which turns the liquid fat into a solid fat and you will see this labelled as 'partially hydrogenated' oil. This type of fat has no health benefits and results in an increase in LDL, the 'bad' cholesterol and a decrease in 'HDL', the 'good' cholesterol. This is the worst combination you can get in terms of the effects on cardiovascular health. Trans fats also occur naturally in ruminant animals and the WHO states that these are thought to have a similar effect on our health as manufactured trans fats.[6] This has led to them advising that less than 1% of our overall energy consumption should come from trans fats. This is the equivalent of around 2.2 g per day for someone eating 2000 kcal.

In addition to our heart health, trans fats have a negative impact on health and fertility in a number of ways. Data from the Nurses Health Study II[7] shows that trans fats found in fast foods, baked goods and other commercially prepared products is associated with an increased risk of infertility for both men and women, and also an increased risk of endometriosis.[6] In men saturated and trans fats are associated with lower semen quality and markers of poor testicular function, and in women the risk of ovulatory infertility is doubled when trans fats are chosen over monounsaturated fats (see below). This may be due to trans fats being associated with inflammation and insulin resistance, both of which are known to impair ovulatory function and make hormone driven conditions more difficult to manage.

You may be wondering why they are used in our food if they have such serious effects on our health and that is also a question I would love to see answered. The main reason is because they prolong the shelf-life of food and are mostly used in baked goods. I would advise you to check the labels and if you see partially hydrogenated oil or PHO in the ingredients, avoid.

Unsaturated fats – Polyunsaturated fatty acids

There are two types of unsaturated fat: monounsaturated fatty acids (MUFAs) and polyunsaturated fatty acids (PUFAs), and individually or together they have been shown to have positive effects on male and female fertility.

PUFAs are otherwise known as omega fatty acids, and are divided into omega-3 and omega-6. The main plant sources are vegetable oils, nuts, seeds, soya and leafy vegetables. There are two essential fatty acids within the PUFA family that cannot be made by the body and must be obtained from the diet: ALA (alpha-linolenic acid, an omega-3) and LA (linoleic acid, an omega-6). While it is easy to consume enough LA on a plant-based diet, it is more challenging to consume enough ALA. This is because ultimately we need our bodies to convert ALA into the usable forms, EPA (eicosapentaenoic acid) and DHA (docosahexaenoic acid) and there are many factors which can inhibit this. Taking a supplement is the easiest way to ensure we are meeting our needs, but this doesn't mean we should neglect our intakes of whole food sources as they contain a range of other important nutrients. The best sources include flaxseeds/linseed, chia seeds, hemp seeds and walnuts. Flaxseeds and hemp should be ground as whole ones pass straight through our digestive system, so although they are a great natural laxative, the nutrients contained in them will not be absorbed sufficiently by your body. Chia seeds are so tiny they can be eaten as they are. Those on a plant-based diet should aim for 2 tbsp daily of any of these seeds. I usually have 1 tbsp of chia and 1 tbsp of flax over the course of the day. I love ground hemp but it isn't always as easy to come by. If you are having the oils, for example flaxseed oil, 1 tbsp a day is enough. Other useful sources of omega-3 if eaten regularly include leafy green vegetables and tofu.

Unfortunately, there are several factors that can interfere with the conversion of ALA into the EPA and DHA, as mentioned above. One factor is if your diet is high in omega-6 foods as omega-6 and omega-3 compete for absorption. If you think of omega-6 as being the tortoise and omega-3 as being the hare, you can work out who wins the competition. Eating large quantities of omega-6 is very common when eating a plant-based diet. Examples of foods with high content include vegetable oils, some nuts and seeds, and oats. Rather than reducing these foods though, you can just add a source of omega-3 foods alongside. So, for example, if you are eating porridge, top it with crushed walnuts and stir in some chia seeds. Similarly, if you are having a smoothie, throw in some chia or flax, or enjoy some dates stuffed with walnut halves.

Other factors that can affect conversion of ALA into DHA and EPA include trans fat intakes (yet another reason to avoid these), caffeine, alcohol, smoking, poor nutritional status, diets very high in overall fat and even your gender. Women of childbearing age convert better than men, which may be due to oestrogen boosting the making of DHA in preparation for pregnancy and lactation.

Protein power smoothie

For those of you who have higher protein needs, a smoothie is a fast and nutritious way of increasing protein intakes without the need for processed protein powders. This is my favourite smoothie made with higher-protein soya milk, fruit, chia seeds and nut butter. It provides 20 g of protein per glass – that's pretty impressive!

- 200 ml plant protein soya milk
- ½ tsp ground turmeric
- ½ tsp ground cinnamon
- 1 tbsp chia seeds
- ½ banana
- Large handful of frozen mixed berries
- 1 tbsp smooth peanut butter
- 1 tbsp cacao

Method
1. Put all the ingredients in a high-speed blender and blend until smooth and thick.
2. Enjoy straight away as the mixture tends to separate if left.

It is well known that omega-3s have anti-inflammatory benefits, but it is a common misconception that omega-6s have the opposite effect and cause inflammation in the body. The theory that omega-6s are pro-inflammatory stems from the fact that LA is converted into arachidonic acid (another type of omega-6) in the body. This is thought to create inflammation, as well as having negative effects on glucose metabolism and weight. However, studies have shown that our bodies regulate arachidonic acid carefully and that higher intakes of LA do not increase levels in our bodies, or increase clinical markers of inflammation.[9]

Omega-3-containing foods may be especially important for male fertility. A randomised controlled trial, the gold standard of all clinical studies, found that supplementing a group of men aged between 21 and 35 years old with 75 g (a higher dose than daily recommendations of 30 g) of walnuts daily for 12 weeks resulted in improved sperm vitality, motility and shape.[10] The control group, who didn't change their diets at all, did not show any improvements in sperm quality. These men were not following a plant-based diet so imagine the results of a trial using a group of fully plant-based men versus a group of men following a standard western diet: I would love to see the outcomes of that study! Interestingly, 75 g of walnuts would provide approximately 6.5 g of ALA, around twice the daily suggested intake for vegans, so this higher quantity may be effective for boosting conversion and may be why this dose was chosen for the study.

A review in 2019 looked at 16 studies that had examined the effects of omega-3 fats or dietary fish intake on semen quality.[11] Four of the studies looked at the effects of omega-3 supplements on sperm quality of men who either had a history of infertility or who were going through tests due to failure to conceive. Three out of the four studies showed that supplementation with either DHA and EPA, or DHA alone, improved at least one fertility marker. These included sperm count, concentration, motility, structure and reduced damage to the sperm DNA (fragmentation). The remaining study did not find any positive effects on sperm quality with supplementation; however, it was a poorer quality study compared to the other three. The fact that these benefits were shown with omega-3 supplements containing EPA and DHA is significant. The supplements were not vegan, but if the effects were from the EPA and DHA, it can be assumed the same effects would be seen with a vegan supplement containing EPA and DHA, both of which are originally found in algae, not fish as explained earlier.

The reason omega-3s are so important for male fertility is because the vast majority of sperm is made up of PUFAs, especially DHA, and the proportion of DHA in sperm increases as the sperm mature. Immature sperm contain about 4% DHA but this increases to about 20% in mature sperm. One study found supplementing with EPA and DHA resulted in higher sperm membrane DHA content, which then resulted in associated higher sperm motility and normal shape and concentration.[12]

For women, the evidence around omega-3s and fertility is less convincing, at least for women trying to conceive naturally without the aid of fertility treatment. There was no association found between higher PUFA intakes and a decreased risk of ovulatory infertility in the Nurses Health Study II, and a recent paper concludes the same.[13]

While studies on natural fertility do not consistently show benefits with omega-3 intakes, the opposite is true for women going through fertility treatment where higher intakes of omega-3 have been associated with higher chances of pregnancy and live birth, as well as improved embryo quality.[12]

When it comes to interpreting the evidence, although there are conflicting outcomes in terms of whether or not PUFAs are beneficial to fertility, the fact that there are associated benefits for men, and for women going through fertility treatment gives grounds for recommending sufficient intakes for all women and couples trying to conceive.

Unsaturated fats – Monounsaturated fatty acids (MUFAs)

The richest source of MUFAs are olives, olive oil, avocados and most nuts. (Walnuts and pine nuts are the exception.)

For women, MUFAs seem to be more important in terms of fertility than PUFAs. Diets higher in MUFAs have been associated with higher fertility rates, and consuming foods rich in this type of fat in place of saturated and trans fats may help to improve fertility. In fact, it has been shown that a Mediterranean diet rich in MUFAs is associated with almost a 70% lower risk of ovulatory infertility when compared with diets high in trans fats.[8] It stands to reason that there will be benefits in replacing trans fats, but that is a pretty impressive statistic. Such a diet is also associated with up to a 90% reduced risk of pre-term delivery.[14]

Studies have also shown that MUFAs play a key role in the development of the foetus. Researchers took blood samples from healthy mothers and their babies to look at their blood fatty-acid profile. The researchers found that MUFAs made up almost a third of the blood fatty acids of the mothers, 18% of the umbilical cord and 23% of the blood of the newborn infant.[15] An earlier study found that MUFA levels were significantly lower in babies who were small for gestational age when compared with babies who were considered a normal weight for gestational age.[16] Although the reasons for this were not clear, it does highlight that MUFAs may play an important role in foetal development.

MUFAs have also been shown to be an important addition to the diet of women going through IVF treatment, with higher intakes associated with nearly a three–and-a-half times higher chance of a live birth after embryo transfer compared with women who had lower intakes.[17]

One food particularly high in MUFAs are avocados. In fact, they make up two thirds of the fatty acid content. Not only that, but they also contain a range of other nutrients essential in the preconception period so they really do make an excellent addition to the diet. These nutrients include folate, choline and vitamins A and E. Avocados have an excellent mix of two different types of fibre, both of which are associated with a lower risk of pre-eclampsia.[14] This is a potentially serious condition marked by excessively high blood pressure that can occur in pregnancy and needs immediate attention. As replacing saturated fats with MUFAs has been shown to improve fertility, avocados can be used to replace butter/

margarine when making sandwiches/toast, and can be blended with garlic and lime juice to create a creamy pasta sauce. To avoid salad dressings with added salt, sugar and preservatives, avocados can be blended with some soya yoghurt, or plant yoghurt of choice, a touch of tahini (leave out if you have a sesame allergy) and a generous twist of black pepper.

Creamy avocado pasta

- 1 ripe avocado, halved with the stone removed
- 1 garlic clove
- Juice of half a lime
- 10 cherry tomatoes
- 75 g whole-wheat pasta per person

Method
1. Cook the pasta as per instructions on the pack.
2. Place the avocado, garlic and lime juice in a small food processor and blend until smooth.
3. When there are two minutes left on the pasta cooking time, add the cherry tomatoes to the pan.
4. Drain the pasta and tomatoes, stir through the sauce, season with salt and pepper and then serve sprinkled with nutritional yeast.

Protein

'But where will I get enough protein?'

This is the most common question I am asked by patients who are considering transitioning to a plant-based diet. Men, in particular those who do a lot of strength training, are always especially concerned about how they are going to meet their protein needs without piling meat onto their plates and whey protein into their post-workout smoothies. The good news is that you will find protein in all plants, there are just some foods that contain much higher amounts than others. For those concerned with their strength gains being compromised, there are a huge number of plant-based athletes, including body builders Nimai Delgado, Korin Sutton and Sam Shorkey, and strongman competitor Patrik Baboumian. There are also a number of current and retired plant-based athletes who are arguably the greatest ever sports people in their discipline, including Lewis Hamilton, Venus Williams, Scott Jurek and Jermain Defoe.

The concerns around protein are in part caused by the many myths circulating on social media and even in national newspapers. A common myth is that plants are not 'complete proteins' – that is, they do not contain all of the nine essential amino acids (so called because your body cannot make these and you need to get them from your diet) needed for your body to build protein. Sceptics continuously use this as an argument not to give up meat, but actually it is factually incorrect. Plants do contain all nine essential amino acids, just in varying amounts. As long as you are eating a varied diet containing whole grains, legumes, lentils, chickpeas, vegetables, fruit, nuts and seeds, and importantly, meeting your energy needs, you will also be meeting your protein needs. Incidentally, soya contains all essential amino acids in a similar proportion to egg white, with tofu containing around 13 g of protein per 100 g and tempeh containing an impressive 21 g, which is equal to the same quantity of steak.

Soya – what's the deal?

Now might be a good time to dispel some of those soya myths, as this is something that comes up time and time again when I speak to patients, and remains rife on social media. A common misconception about soya is that, because of its phytoestrogen content, it can alter hormone production, in particular testosterone in men, thereby leading to 'feminisation'. However, a recent review of over 40 studies found no association at all between soya and negative impacts on male hormone levels, or sexual function,[18] and this means it is also completely safe to give to male babies and children. I have been giving my son soya milk practically since birth, and more recently tofu several times a week, and have no qualms about doing so.

Another concern is that soya is associated with reduced ovarian reserves. This is due to some small studies suggesting it may negatively impact blood FSH levels, a measurement that was used as a marker of ovarian reserve. However, the studies were not similar in design and did not use more accurate measures of ovarian reserve, such as anti-Müllerian hormone (AMH) levels. Furthermore, if soya does have this effect, we would expect to see women with higher intakes reach menopause earlier and no such associations have been found. For women undergoing fertility treatment, soya has been associated with a higher probability of live birth, thicker endometrial tissue and successful pregnancy.[19]

A recent review of the effects of soya and soya isoflavones on women's fertility and related outcomes agreed with this and concluded that it is possible that soya improves outcomes for women going through fertility treatment and may benefit women with endocrine disorders, including PCOS and endometriosis.[20] By the way, soya and 'soy' are exactly the same thing; they just are different spellings depending on the country. For example, it is spelled 'soya' in the UK and Europe, and 'soy' in America and Australia.

Tofu is my absolute favourite soya product because it is so tasty and so versatile, but the key to a great tofu dish rather than a mediocre dish is in the preparation.

Creamy tofu curry

- 1 block of tofu, pressed and cut into medium cubes
- 1 tin of tomatoes
- 1 onion
- 3 cloves of garlic
- 1 heaped tsp each of turmeric and garam masala
- 2 tsp ground cumin
- ½ tsp ground fenugreek
- 1 inch piece of ginger, grated
- ½ vegetable stock cube
- 4 tbsp soya Greek-style yoghurt
- Handful of fresh coriander, roughly chopped

Method
1. Chop the onion and sauté either in olive oil or water/ vegetable stock until soft.
2. Chop the garlic then add to the pan with the ginger and cook for 2-3 minutes.
3. Add the spices and stir until lovely and fragrant.
4. Add the tomatoes plus ¼ of the can of water, the stock cube and the tofu.
5. Bring to the boil then reduce and simmer with the lid on for 25 minutes.
6. Stir through the yoghurt and coriander, then serve with brown rice.

Tempeh is also excellent but you need to prepare it in a slightly different way. It can be quite bitter but I find this disappears if you steam it in a little water for 10 minutes before marinading and cooking. You don't need a fancy steamer; just a little water in a pan with the lid on works a treat. If you haven't tried it yet, give it a go. It has a different texture to tofu; it's much firmer and has the added bonus of being a fermented food so your gut bacteria will love it. Unlike tofu though, you must cook it before eating to avoid the risk of bacteria-borne illnesses. I find that tempeh is a marmite food – that is, you either really like it or really dislike it. It may appeal to males as the texture is similar to meat and it has more substance than tofu. Personally, I enjoy it but in moderation; I'm definitely more a tofu kind of girl and could happily eat it for lunch and dinner every day (and some days I do!) Smoked tofu is always a regular part of my diet as it is such a simple way to increase the protein content of your lunch. You don't need to cook it, heat it or marinade; you can simply slice and add it to sandwiches/wraps/pittas, or cut it into cubes and throw these on top of a mixed salad with some avocado and a drizzle of balsamic vinegar. Delicious!

Table 4: Protein content per serving of a variety of plant foods

Food	Serving size	Protein (g)
Legumes		
Beans (black, black-eyed, kidney, pinto, cannellini, chickpeas)	90 g	6-7
Lentils (red, green, brown puy)	80 g	5-7
Peanut butter (100% peanuts)	30 g	9

Peanuts	30 g	8
Peas (frozen)	50 g	3
Soybeans	50 g	7
Soya milk	200 ml	6-10
Tempeh	80 g	10-13
Tofu (medium-firm or firm)	80 g	10
Grains (uncooked)		
Oats	40 g	4
Quinoa	50 g	3.5
Rice (brown/red/black)	75 g	7
Rice (white)	75 g	7
Wholewheat pasta	75 g	10
White pasta	75 g	10
Wholewheat couscous	50 g	7
Wholemeal bread	1 medium slice	4
Wholemeal bagel	1 bagel	9.6
White bread	1 medium slice	3.5
Buckwheat	40 g	3
Nuts, seeds and butters		
Almonds, cashews	30 g	6
Pecans	30 g	3
Pistachios	30 g	7
Walnuts	30 g	5
Chia seeds, flax seeds (ground)	30 g	7
Pumpkin/sesame/sunflower seeds	30 g	6-7
Almond butter – 100% almonds	30 g	8

Table 4: Protein content Cont'd

Food	Serving size	Protein (g)
Tahini	30 g	7.5
Vegetables (raw)		
Avocado	80 g	1.5
Broccoli	80 g	3
Cauliflower	80 g	2
Sweetcorn	80 g	2
Carrot	80 g	0.4
Kale	80 g	2.7
Potato	1 medium	4
Sweet potato	1 medium	2.5
Butternut squash	200 g	2
Green beans	80 g	1.7
Chestnut mushrooms	100 g	1
Fruit (raw)		
Apple/pear	1 typical size	0.5
Banana	1 medium	1.8
Mango	100 g	0.7
Orange	1 typical size	1
Blueberries	80 g	0.7
Strawberries	100 g	0.8
Raspberries	80 g	1
Dates	30 g	0.6
Fortified milks and yoghurts		
Soya milk	100 ml	3
Protein power soya milk	100 ml	5
Soya yoghurt	125 g	5-6
Miscellaneous		
Nutritional yeast	5 g	2.4

As you can see from Table 4, protein is everywhere, even in fruit and vegetables. It is true that the protein contents of fruit and vegetables are much lower than other plant foods but when eaten daily they make useful contributions. For example, adding in some avocado, mushrooms and green beans to a tofu-based dish will increase the protein content of your meal by around 4 g.

You can use Table 5 (page 141) to ensure that you are meeting your protein needs daily (see below). However, it isn't generally something that is a concern as long as you are meeting your daily energy needs. Again, these vary depending on your age, activity levels, weight and gender but your body is very good at regulating how much energy you need as long as you let it guide you. The problems arise when meals are based around carbohydrates – for example, pasta and sauce without adding beans or tofu or chickpeas, or when breakfast cereal is chosen without the addition of nuts and seeds, so it is really important to ensure a good source of protein with every meal and snack. Protein is vital for health. Our tissues need it to grow, for maintenance and for repair. It is vital for optimum immune function and for our bodies to heal from injury and inflammation, among many other things. So, ensuring you get enough in your diet is important, but that is the case for all eating patterns, not just those following a plant-based diet.

When it comes to protein requirements, there is a bit of a debate about whether plant-based eaters need slightly more than meat eaters due to the high fibre of plant foods reducing absorption. Guidelines for protein vary between 0.7 and 0.8 g per kilogram of body weight (g/kg) depending on where you are in the world, but I always recommend 1 gram per kilogram (1 g/kg) of protein as a basic rule for any dietary pattern. This does vary depending on your age, the amount and type of physical activity you do, and/or any underlying medical conditions where your protein needs are higher. If you exercise moderately you do not actually need to increase your protein intake. This really applies to people who do cardio or strength training for several hours each week, which takes the threshold above moderate exercise. As I will explain later, I would not recommend men or women trying to conceive to do regular, strenuous exercise, but for those individuals protein needs vary between 1.2 and 1.7 grams per kilogram of body weight per day (g/kg-bw/day). There is very little evidence to suggest intakes above this range are beneficial.

To show you how easy it is to meet even much higher protein needs, let's take the example of an 87 kg male who combines a mix of cardio and intense strength training weekly. He has chosen to set his protein needs at 1.7 g/kg-bw/day, meaning he aims to eat 148 g of protein daily. The box shows an example of how he can meet those needs with food alone and no protein supplements.

How an 87 kg man meets his protein needs in a day

Breakfast: Porridge (50-60 g oats as the standard portion size will not be enough for increased energy needs) made with higher-protein soya milk, topped with chia seeds, pumpkin seeds, walnuts, peanut butter, mixed berries and banana.

Snack: Wholemeal bagel with almond butter, milled hemp seeds and blueberries.

Lunch: Jacket potato with beans and nutritional yeast, side salad with tahini dressing. Greek-style soya yoghurt.

Snack: Homemade smoothie (see smoothie receipe, page 124) and 10 almonds.

Dinner: Baked tofu with brown rice, sweetcorn, kale and sesame seeds, with avocado sauce.

Evening snack: Two oat cakes with hummous and sesame seeds. Satsuma.

MICRONUTRIENTS ESSENTIAL FOR FERTILITY

Folate and folic acid (vitamin B9)

It was almost 60 years ago that the link between folate deficiency and pregnancy complications was first observed,[23] and it is now well known that women considering pregnancy and also those in their first trimester of pregnancy should be taking a 400 mcg of folic acid supplement to reduce the risk of neural tube defects (NTDs – spina bifida is the best known).

A woman's folate needs increase during pregnancy due to several changes, including enlargement of the uterus and the development of the placenta so it is vital that her folate stores are plentiful. We don't really know why folic acid prevents NTDs but many studies have shown supplementation is associated with a fourfold reduced risk of an NTD-affected pregnancy and also recurrence if a previous pregnancy has been affected.[24] Folic acid supplementation is also associated with a reduced risk of low birth weight, heart defects and pre-term birth.[24] Folate (vitamin B9 in its natural form) and folic acid (B9 in its synthetic form) are not just essential during pregnancy though; they are also really important during the pre-conception period, especially as many women do not know they are pregnant in the very early stages of pregnancy. By the time some women realise they are pregnant, it may be too late to start taking folic acid as the neural tube closes by around week four of pregnancy and any problems will have already happened. There are no clear guidelines about when to start taking folic acid, but I would say it is sensible to start taking it at least three months before you start trying for a baby or start fertility treatment.

Can all women take folic acid?

Folic acid guidelines apply to all women, even for those known to have one or two 'MTHFR variants'. MTHFR stands for methylene-tetrahydrofolate reductase and a variant basically means your body cannot process folate as quickly. You may have read that taking folic acid will be ineffective if you have one or two variants in MTHFR but this is not true. Taking folic acid at the recommended 400 mcg a day will still significantly help you to reduce the risk of neural tube defects (NTDs). There is another folate supplement called 5-MTHFR but the problem is there are no studies to show that this has the same protective effect as folic acid so guidance cannot be given.

For women going through IVF, there is evidence that folic acid supplementation may improve the outcomes of treatment.[25]

Miscarriage concerns

There was some concern about folic acid supplementation in the early 1990s when a few studies suggested that it was associated with an increased risk of miscarriage. However, many large studies and reviews of studies since that time have found there to be no association,[26] even with higher doses of 4 mg daily, and actually data from large studies, including the Nurses Health Study II, suggest a lower risk of miscarriage among women taking folic acid prior to or during the first trimester at higher doses than the current guidelines for the prevention of NTDs.

Some women need more

Although the recommendation for folic acid is 400 mcg a day for most women and, in some countries, up to 800 mcg, some will need a much higher dose of 5 mg, and this can only be prescribed by a doctor. In the UK, NICE recommend that 5 mg will be needed if either partner has a NTD, or there is a history of NTDs in the family, or there has been a previous pregnancy affected by a NTD. You will also have to take a higher dose if you are on anti-epileptic medication, if you have diabetes and certain other conditions, or if you have a BMI above 30 kg/m^2. If you fall into any of these categories, or if you are concerned, it is important that you discuss this with your doctor before you start trying to conceive so that you are taking the correct dose.

Male needs

Folate is also important for men as it is needed to produce the DNA in sperm. Studies have shown significant improvement in sperm counts when infertile men were given folic acid and zinc supplements,[25] as well as improvements in sperm concentration and shape.[26] However, a recent randomised clinical trial looking at 2370 men planning on undergoing fertility treatment with their female partners did not find any significant differences in sperm parameters or live birth between men who were supplemented with 5 mg of folic acid and 30 mg of zinc for six months and those who did not receive supplements.[27] In fact, there was a higher incidence of sperm DNA damage in the supplemented group and also some mild gastrointestinal side effects. This may be a result of the zinc dose far exceeding the daily requirement for men. Higher doses of zinc are associated with gastrointestinal side effects and there is the risk of zinc toxicity if taken for long periods of time. The reason the men were supplemented with zinc as well as folate was because they work synergistically together – that is, folate and zinc work together to increase the amounts entering the bloodstream to have a more active effect. Zinc is also approximately 30 times higher in seminal fluid than in blood, suggesting a link to semen quality, and this may be because of its antioxidant properties. However, as with all vitamins and minerals, taking high doses via a supplement is not recommended and ensuring optimum dietary intake should be the focus.

Although there is insufficient evidence to advise men to take a folic acid supplement in the same way as women, good dietary folate intake is essential and it is abundant in a plant-based diet. See Table 5 opposite for sources and requirements for men and women during preconception and pregnancy.

Our bodies also need folate in order to produce healthy red blood cells and lower the risk of anaemia, so ensuring you have adequate folate intakes is just as important as ensuring you are eating enough iron-rich food. If you are deficient in folate, there is the risk of a particular type of anaemia called megaloblastic anaemia. This is when your red blood cells are bigger than normal and also fewer, and their size means they may not be able to leave your bone marrow to enter the bloodstream and deliver oxygen. The developing baby is to some extent protected from this as they will draw from their mother's folate stores, but there is evidence that if their mother does not take in sufficient folate during pregnancy, there is the risk of low birth weight which then increases the risk of developmental and long-term health effects.[28]

Some women have asked me if they need to take a folic acid supplement if they are eating plenty of folate-rich foods and the answer is YES! It is easy to imagine that you will continue to eat sufficient dietary folate if you are eating plenty of folate-rich foods at the moment, but the picture may well be very different if you fall pregnant. The first trimester often brings bouts of morning sickness, which can be severe in some women. If you've experienced a stomach bug where you've felt very nauseas or have been sick you will remember having no appetite and feeling queasy at the very thought of eating. Can you imagine trying to work your way through a plate of leafy greens and brown rice? The likelihood is that all you felt like eating once the worst was over was plain toast, or crackers, or ginger biscuits to try and combat the nausea. This is a common diet for many women in the first trimester of pregnancy and it is not going to provide the folate needed to help protect against NTDs.

Table 5: Example micronutrient sources and requirements for men, and women for preconception and pregnancy.[46, 47, 48]

Micro-nutrient	Recommended nutrient intake (RNI)/accept-able intakes (AI)	Example food sources	Portion size	Content
Vitamin B9: folate	Unit: mcg Men – 400 Preconception – 400 Pregnancy – 600 Women should take a 400 mcg or 5 mg folic acid supplement during precon-ception and pregnancy	Spinach Avocado Banana Grapefruit Kiwi Orange Beetroot Broccoli Walnuts Seeds Quinoa Rye bread Wholewheat bread Weetabix Fortified nutri-tional yeast	30 g ½ medium 1 medium ½ medium 1 medium 1 large 120 g 80 g (cooked) 30 g 30 g 100 g (cooked) 1 slice 1 slice 2 bix 5 g	58 81 24 16 19 55 78 85 28 25 40 45 14 64 220
Vitamin B12: cobala-min	Unit: mcg Men – 3 Women – 3 Preconception – 3 Pregnancy – 3 Both genders should take a 25-50 mcg sup-plement daily	Fortified nutri-tional yeast Marmite Fortified plant milk Fortified break-fast cereal	5 g 8 g 100 ml 30 g	2.2 1.9 0.38 0.63
Vitamin A	Unit: mcg Men – 900 Women – 700 Preconception – 700 Pregnancy – 770	Cantaloupe melon Grapefruit Red bell pepper Carrot Cooked, mashed sweet potato	1 medium slice 1 medium 1 medium 1 medium 100 g	139 143 186 510 1,364

Micro-nutrient	Recommended nutrient intake (RNI)/accept-able intakes (AI)	Example food sources	Portion size	Content
Vitamin C	Unit: mg Men – 40 Women – 40 Preconception – 40 Pregnancy - 50	Apple Orange Kiwi Pear Avocado Carrot Red bell pepper Tomato	1 medium 1 medium 1 medium 1 medium ½ medium 1 medium ½ medium 1 medium	8 70 70 7 10 4 75 17
Vitamin D	Unit: mcg Men - 15 Women – 15 Preconception – 15 Pregnancy – 15 Both genders should take a 10-50 mcg sup-plement during the winter months and for some all year round	Fortified milk Fortified cereal Fortified yoghurt Sunbathed mushrooms	100 ml 30 g 100 g 100 g	0.75-1 0.8-2.5 0.75-1.1 1.5
Vitamin E	Unit: mg Men – 11 Women - 11 Preconception – 11 Pregnancy - 11	Avocado Dried apricots Kiwi Red bell pepper Almond butter Peanut butter Almonds Sunflower seeds	½ medium 30 g 1 medium ½ medium 2 tbsp 2 tbsp 30 g 30 g	2.1 2.6 1.1 1 8 2.9 4.8 3.7
Selenium	Unit: mcg Men – 70 Women – 70 Preconception – 70 Pregnancy – 70	Mushrooms Chia seeds Brazil nuts Kidney beans Calcium-set tofu	50 g 30 g 30 g 100 g 100 g	5 18 680 100 10-18

Zinc	Unit: mg Men – 11 Women – 8 Preconception – 8 Pregnancy – 11	Almond butter Almonds Hemp seeds Chia seeds Sesame seeds Sunflower seeds Oats Quinoa Wholewheat bread	2 tbsp 30 g 30 g 30 g 30 g 30 g 50 g 50 g 1 slice	1.1 1.1 2 1.7 2.5 1.5 1.2 1.1 0.5
Iodine	Unit: mcg Men – 150 Women – 150 Preconception – 150 Pregnancy – 200 Both genders should take a 150 mcg supplement daily	The only reliable source when on a plant-based diet is a daily supplement		
Iron	Unit: mg Men – 11 Women – 16 Preconception – 16 Pregnancy – 16	Avocado Kale Cooked peas Baked potato Seeds Nuts Legumes Calcium-set tofu	1 medium 65 g 65 g 1 medium 30 g 30 g 40 g 100 g	1.1 1-2 1.3 1.9 2-5 1-3 2-3.5 1.7-3
Choline	Unit: mg Men – 400 Women – 400 Preconception – 400 Pregnancy – 480	Edamame beans Shiitake mushrooms (cooked) Potato (red) Quinoa (cooked) Broccoli (cooked) Brown rice (cooked)	100 145 g 1 large 180 g 90 g 250 g	214 118 57 43 31 19

Vitamin B12

It is well known that those following a plant-based diet should be supplementing B12. It is theoretically possible to achieve adequate B12 via fortified foods, but this needs careful planning and there are many situations where it might not be possible. For example, if you are on holiday, going away for the weekend, or have lost your appetite as a result of illness. It is for these reasons and more that I always recommend a daily 25-50 mcg supplement. You can take a larger dose of 2000 mcg once a week, or split it into 2 x 1000 mcg, but the problem with that is you may well forget. Taking a supplement daily is much easier to remember and will ensure you do not become deficient as long as you do not have any absorption issues. If you look at the daily requirements for B12 you will see that they are only 2.4 mcg a day so you may be wondering why I recommend a much higher dose. The answer to that is our bodies can only absorb a small amount of B12 at one time, so even if you were to take a 2.4 mcg supplement, not all of it would be absorbed. The best way to make sure that your body absorbs enough B12 is to take a higher dose supplement, and 25-50 mcg is sufficient for most people.

Many of those on a plant-based diet use nutritional yeast regularly as a source of B12 and I would encourage this as it also contains some protein and a range of other nutrients. Relying on it solely for B12, however, is not a good idea because you would have to eat an awful lot of it to get 25 mcg: 55 g in fact, which is a huge undertaking, even if you have a 'nooch' obsession (like me!).

Although signs of B12 deficiency can take years to manifest, (so you don't need to panic if you are new to plant-based eating and have not yet started supplementing), they can be serious and include fatigue, depression, anaemia and nervous system damage. It can also lead to megaloblastic anaemia in the same way as folate deficiency. One of the early signs of B12 deficiency can be tingling in your hands and feet, but if left untreated it can ultimately cause irreversible brain damage. This is why, even if you are taking a daily supplement, it is a good idea to have an annual blood test to check your B12 levels if you are following a plant-based diet. This will also help your doctor identify if you have problems absorbing B12 because, if your levels are low despite supplementing correctly, you may be deficient in something called intrinsic factor. This is a protein excreted by the stomach to enable you to absorb B12. If this is the case, you will need regular B12 injections to ensure sufficient levels.

The role of B12 in male and female fertility

In men, low B12 blood levels are associated with infertility because there are effects on sperm concentration, motility and shape, and damage to the DNA.[29]

In women, low blood levels are linked to recurrent miscarriage, an increased risk of pre-eclampsia, and infertility. In contrast, sufficient levels have been shown to increase mature egg quantity and improve embryo quality. B12 also helps us to absorb folic acid, so a deficiency pre-pregnancy could increase the risk of NTDs, and it could also risk deficiency in the newborn.[28] You can probably detect a running theme here that nutrients very rarely act alone; they are often dependent on one or more other nutrients to act effectively.

The overriding message I want to get across here is that relying on fortified foods for your B12 is not enough. You must take a supplement to ensure you do not become deficient. There are also certain groups who are at higher risk of deficiency and these include:

- Those on certain medications that affect absorption of the vitamin. These include some medications prescribed for reflux or other conditions, certain antibiotics, some cholesterol-lowering drugs and some diabetes medications.
- Those with inflammatory bowel disease, especially poorly controlled coeliac disease, and those who have undergone

surgery on their bowel, particularly the small intestine as this is where B12 is absorbed.

All of these groups will be able to have B12 injections if necessary, so if you are concerned please do speak with your doctor.

To reassure you though, if you fit into the 'general population' bracket, where you are fit and healthy and are not on certain long-term medications, and you are consuming fortified foods and taking a daily supplement in the correct dose, it really is extremely rare to be B12 deficient.

Vitamin A

Vitamin A is a fat-soluble vitamin that has many roles, including in reproduction, DNA synthesis and protection, normal development of the embryo, and eye health and a healthy immune system in the baby.[14] Vitamin A also plays an important part in sperm health, as it may help to regulate their shape and concentration.

Higher blood levels of vitamin A have been found in men with normal sperm parameters compared with men with oligospermia (low sperm count), asthenozoospermia (reduced sperm motility) and azoospermia (absence of sperm). However, supplementation increases the risk of consuming too much vitamin A and long-term, excessive intake may negatively affect sperm production, shape, motility and viability.[29] This is why I do not recommend vitamin A supplements to my male patients and will always advise the 'food first' approach.

Different forms of vitamin A

There are two forms of vitamin A: preformed from animal products, and provitamin A from some colourful plant foods. These colourful pigments are called carotenoids and you may have heard of beta-carotene, one of the most commonly known carotenoids. Examples of fruit and vegetables containing beta-carotene include cantaloupe melon, mango, butternut squash, carrots and sweet potato. Once you eat these fruit and vegetables your body will convert the carotenoids into the active form of vitamin A known as retinol. There are other carotenoids, including lycopene, which are in the red fruit and vegetables, such as tomatoes and watermelon, but they cannot be converted into vitamin A. They do, however, have other health and fertility benefits, so red fruit and vegetables should certainly be a regular part of your diet.

Two key carotenoids for a baby's eye health while in the womb are called lutein and zeaxanthin, and while they are either not present in or well absorbed from many fruit and vegetables, they are contained in significant amounts in avocados. The key factor here is the fat content of this fruit, as carotenoids are better absorbed with a source of fat. As avocados also contain beta-carotene, which can be converted into vitamin A, they really are an excellent addition to the diet for both pregnant women and also women trying to conceive.

Studies have shown that if you eat a salad with carotenoid-containing vegetables, for example grated carrot, cooked and cubed squash and/or sweet potato, and it also contains avocado, the absorption of those carotenoids and subsequent vitamin A conversion is increased by up to 15 times compared with a salad without avocado.[14] The same effect may be achievable by drizzling olive oil on your salad, and this is absolutely fine, but it's worth bearing in mind that, although extra virgin olive oil has been shown to have many health benefits and is of course a significant addition to the healthful Mediterranean-style diet, it does not contain many of the fertility-friendly nutrients of an avocado. If you are preparing a salad I would always recommend throwing in some avocado first, and then, if you have made an olive oil-based dressing, you can always drizzle that over the top.

Although ensuring adequate dietary vitamin A is essential during preconception for both men and women, and in pregnancy, women trying to conceive should not take a supplement containing preformed vitamin A. This is because excessive amounts are associated with miscarriage and congenital defects involving the nervous and cardiovascular systems. This same reasoning applies to animal sources rich in vitamin A, including liver, liver patés and cod liver oil supplements.

How to get enough vitamin A from a plant-based diet

I often come across myths about our body's ability to convert carotenoids into retinol, with those unfamiliar with plant-based diets and human anatomy claiming we cannot convert plant foods into vitamin A efficiently. As is usually the case though, these claims are unfounded. As long as you are eating a range of fruit and vegetables daily, paired with a fat source when eaten as part of a meal or a snack, you will easily meet or even exceed your needs.

I have to tell you about one of my favourite way to add the right fats to my meals: tahini. Honestly, it is probably one of the most diverse foods in a plant-based diet as it goes with pretty much anything. If I make a rice dish, I dip my fork in tahini and drizzle it over the top. It is completely delicious over roasted butternut squash, carrots and sweet potato. If you haven't tried this you must – it will change your life! You can also add a teaspoon to your porridge at breakfast, along with a couple of chopped dates to sweeten and a teaspoon of cacao powder. You can even bake it into cookies, or just spread it on toast and top with a sprinkle of nutritional yeast.

Other ways to add predominantly unsaturated fats to meals to increase carotenoid absorption include sprinkling pumpkin seeds over sweet potato mash, or chopping some persimmon fruit or mango into your porridge or overnight oats. This tastes even better when you stir through some almond butter.

Just remember that if you do not eat enough fat, your hormone production will be affected, you will feel fatigued, and you will not absorb enough fat-soluble vitamins, including vitamin A. This also applies if you have a medical condition which means you do not absorb fat properly. It is so important to include a source of fat with your meals and to ensure you see your GP if you notice any signs of fat malabsorption, such as unintentional weight loss and/or diarrhoea that is pale or yellow in colour, which floats, and is particularly offensive in smell, or is difficult to flush.

Spiced sweet potato and butternut squash soup

- 1 medium butternut squash, peeled and cut into chunks
- 2 x large sweet potatoes, peeled and cut into chunks
- 2 x onions, chopped roughly
- 1 tsp turmeric
- 1 tsp cumin
- 1 tsp garam masala
- ½ tsp fenugreek
- 2 inch piece of ginger, peeled and grated
- 750 ml vegetable stock
- Handful of roughly chopped coriander
- Juice of half a lemon

Method
1. Sauté the onions and ginger in a little vegetable stock/oil until soft.
2. Stir in the spices and coat the onions.
3. Add the sweet potato and butternut squash and stir well into the onions.
4. Cook for 5 minutes.

5. Add the stock, lemon juice and a little more water if needed so that all the vegetables are just covered.
6. Bring to the boil and then simmer with the lid on for 20 minutes.
7. Transfer in batches to a blender, add the coriander and blend until smooth.
8. Add a twist of black pepper to each bowl and enjoy!

Vitamin C

Vitamin C is a powerful antioxidant, meaning that it can help prevent damage to our cells and DNA, but as we cannot make it in our bodies (like guinea pigs and some primates), we need to consume it as part of our diet. Because of its antioxidant properties, it can help to protect sperm and eggs from the damage caused by oxidative stress, and it also increases iron absorption so it is a really important part of the diet for everyone trying to conceive.

Vitamin C is associated with healthy sperm as when a male consumes enough from food it leads to increases in his semen. This is important as it has been shown to protect the DNA in sperm from damage. Interestingly, semen levels of vitamin C can be 10 times higher than vitamin C in the blood, and may account for 65% of antioxidant activity in the semen.[30] This promotes a healthy environment for sperm to grow and develop and is associated with improved sperm count, motility and shape, and overall fertility.

In women, dietary vitamin C intake has been associated with more antioxidant activity within the ovarian follicles,[31] so it may give more protection to the developing eggs. Higher dietary intakes have also been associated with improved egg maturation and fertilisation.[32]

As with most nutrients, and as supported by the evidence, I recommend that vitamin C should always be consumed via dietary sources rather than supplements as our needs can be met with just one orange a day. Of course, it is best to eat a variety of fruit and vegetables to get your vitamin C, and as they are such rich sources, you certainly don't need to take a supplement. In fact, you can experience adverse reactions from high-strength vitamin C supplements, including stomach cramps, nausea and diarrhoea. There is also the possibility of its role being flipped with very high doses, where instead of acting as an antioxidant it may act as a pro-oxidant. This means it can cause damage rather than protect against it, and at high doses it has been reported to negatively affect oocyte quality.[32] You don't need to worry if your diet is full of vitamin C-containing foods; these effects are only associated with high-dose vitamin C supplements where that single dose is taken in one go without the additional nutrients and fibre found in whole foods. So you can continue to happily aim for as many fruits and vegetables as you can manage.

Vitamin D

Vitamin D is commonly known as the 'sunshine vitamin' as during the summer months most of us can make sufficient amounts via direct sunlight with the help of our skin, liver and kidneys to keep our blood levels topped up without the need for supplementation. When the autumn nights start drawing in, however, the sun's rays are not strong enough for us to make enough vitamin D and everyone should start to take a supplement every day as per the current guidelines. Current guidelines in the UK are 10 mcg a day, but I actually recommend slightly higher than this as global recommendations vary between 10 and 50 mcg per day to maintain blood levels. The Vegan Society has changed its VEG1 supplement formula to account for this, with vitamin D increased from 10 to 20 mcg.

Some people will need to take a supplement all year around and these include:

- those who spend a lot of time indoors.
- people will darker skin who absorb less vitamin D due to higher amounts of melanin in their skin.
- those who wear clothes that cover most of their skin.
- those who have an underlying medical condition or take medications that may change the way vitamin D is absorbed.

I do advise everyone to ask their GP to check their vitamin D levels as deficiency is actually quite common, with about one in five people not having adequate levels. If you are found to have a deficiency, you will need to be prescribed a higher dose supplement than you can buy over the counter until your levels are normal, and then you should be able to maintain with a standard dose.

Vitamin D has two main forms, D2 and D3, and both are absorbed well in the gut. However, D3 is the form naturally produced by our skins in sunlight and is preferable. For this reason, most supplements will contain D3. It used to be the case that you could not get a vegan D3 as supplements used to be made using the form derived from sheep's wool. However, it can now be derived from lichen, which has made it possible to have a vegan vitamin D3 supplement. As vitamin D is fat soluble, I always advise taking your supplement with a meal or snack containing a source of fat as this will help your body absorb it better.

As well as taking a vitamin D supplement during the winter, and for some all year around, and getting adequate, safe sun exposure without burning, it is important to try and eat food sources of vitamin D regularly. One way you can do this is by 'sunbathing' mushrooms, although you can buy them pre-sunbathed. You do this by lining them up either on a sheet outside or on your window sill, upside down to increase the surface area, and they start to make vitamin D just as our skin does; they are incredibly clever! One thing to note is that the rays we need to make vitamin D, UVB rays, cannot penetrate glass, so if you are putting your mushrooms on your window sill make sure you open the window, otherwise your efforts will be in vain. Unfortunately, the skin damaging rays, UVA rays, can penetrate glass, so if you are driving, or sitting in a conservatory or somewhere similar, even on a cloudy day, remember to protect your skin with a high SPF sun cream, especially on your face.

Other useful sources of vitamin D on a plant-based diet are fortified milks and yoghurts and fortified breakfast cereals.

Vitamin D has several functions, including helping us to absorb of calcium, and without adequate intakes our bones would become thin and brittle. In terms of fertility though, vitamin D plays an equally vital role. Men and women have receptors for vitamin D throughout their reproductive system, including in the testes, ovaries, uterus and placenta, and this suggests a need for the vitamin for reproductive health.

Studies looking at vitamin D and sperm parameters have reported conflicting outcomes. Adequate vitamin D levels are associated with normal sperm motility and shape and circulating testosterone levels, but both deficiency and excess vitamin D have negative associations. These include disruptions to sex hormones, including testosterone,[30] and reduced sperm quality, including poorer motility and reduced concentration.[32] However, the degree of vitamin D deficiency appears to be key. Severe deficiency is associated with a range of negative effects on sperm, but mild deficiency (the most common degree of deficiency in the UK), where levels are just below the normal range, appears to have less of an effect, with the main association being reduced motility.[34]

Studies have looked at supplementing men with vitamin D to see whether this improves sperm parameters. One clinical trial showed that, when 330 deficient men were supplemented with vitamin D and also calcium, although there was no difference in sperm concentration, the number of spontaneous pregnancies was higher in the supplemented group than the group who were given a placebo. In another study where men were supplemented with vitamin D and calcium, the sperm count and motility increased, along with an increase in spontaneous pregnancies and testosterone concentrations.[33]

In terms of female fertility, data show that live birth rates for women going through fertility treatment are higher in those with sufficient vitamin D levels.[33] While further clinical trials are needed, I would advise all women, along with their partners if applicable, to get their vitamin D levels checked prior to starting fertility treatment.

Vitamin E

Vitamin E is another fat-soluble vitamin and a vital antioxidant that may play a part in helping to increase the number of mature eggs for collection. It may improve embryo quality in women undergoing IVF treatment.[35] In men the vitamin may promote healthy reproductive function. Sperm are made up of proteins, cholesterol and fats, and are surrounded by a membrane. Vitamin E protects the fats in the membrane and the structure or shape of the sperm. Adequate dietary vitamin E is associated with fertility and normal sperm parameters, and although some trials have shown improved sperm motility with vitamin E and selenium supplements, there is not enough evidence to support routine supplementation and actually there are a number of risks associated with vitamin E supplements.

If you search the internet for vitamin E supplements, the dose range is most commonly 400-1000 international units (IU) per capsule. This equates to 268 mg and 670 mg respectively. Compare this to our daily requirements, which are just 15 mg for both women and men of reproductive age and you can see just how much more you would be taking with a supplement. High doses of 400 IU a day, or long-term use, are associated with an increased risk of heart failure, an increased risk of a brain bleed in men, and an increased risk of prostate cancer, as well as nausea, stomach cramps and diarrhoea. They can also interact with some medications, including blood thinning medications, some statins, and potentially chemotherapy and radiation treatments. They are also associated with increased abdominal pain in pregnancy.[36]

Another consideration is that vitamin E is a fat-soluble vitamin, which means that, unlike water-soluble vitamins, any excess is not removed from your body in your urine. The vitamin is instead stored in your liver and fatty tissues and excess levels can easily build up if you regularly supplement. Being fat-soluble also technically means that you do not need to meet your requirements every day as your body can take what it needs from its stores. However, I do recommend that you still include sources in your diet daily as all foods containing vitamin E are useful sources of the unsaturated fats needed for fertility. Unlike supplements, research has not found any risks to health associated with dietary sources of vitamin E, so you can eat foods including avocadoes, nuts, seeds, fruit and vegetables without concern, and vegetable oils if you choose to include these in your diet.

Selenium

Selenium is a trace element and is important for both male and female fertility. The majority of it is stored in your muscle and deficiency is associated with male infertility.[37] Similarly, in women, levels of selenium in follicular fluid (the fluid that surrounds the developing egg) have been found to be lower in women with unexplained fertility, compared to women who struggle to conceive due to fallopian tube defects.[37] When comparing pregnant women who are deficient in selenium with women who have adequate levels, there has been shown to be an approximate eight times higher risk of pre-term delivery.[28]

Selenium acts as an antioxidant, and may play a part in follicle growth and maturation, protecting the dominant follicle from damage from oxidative stress, and protecting both the sperm and the embryo from oxidative stress. It can be found in high concentrations in the testes and may play a part in sperm motility and viability and overall male fertility.[37]

It is very simple to get adequate amounts of selenium in a plant-based diet. The easiest way to do this is to eat 1-2 Brazil nuts daily, which will enable you to meet your full daily requirements. Grains, legumes and some fruit and vegetables also contain good amounts of selenium. However, to show the difference in selenium content between Brazil nuts and one type of whole grain, brown rice, 1-2 Brazil nuts contain 136-182 mcg of selenium, while a portion of brown rice (60 g, dry weight) contains roughly 10 mcg. When you then look at our daily needs, which are 60 mcg for women and 75 mcg for men, you can appreciate how rich in selenium Brazil nuts are. You should avoid eating more than two in a day, though, as you risk selenium toxicity which can cause symptoms such as nausea, diarrhoea, fatigue, irritability, hair and nail loss, nervous system abnormalities, a metallic taste in your mouth and garlic breath. It is not necessary to supplement with selenium if you enjoy Brazil nuts, but if you are taking a supplement that does contain selenium, I would avoid eating the nuts on a regular basis and just check the supplement dose. Some can contain 200 mcg which is too much.

Zinc

Zinc is another important mineral for both male and female fertility, but it is especially important for men. Why? Because their needs are slightly higher than women's as they lose zinc in each ejaculate. If you are trying for a baby the male has the potential to lose quite a bit! The fact that zinc levels in seminal fluid are so much higher than in blood also points to this micronutrient playing a key role in sperm health.

Zinc also has an important role in testicular development and in sperm maturation. Deficiency is related to low serum testosterone levels in men, and reduced ability of the sperm to fertilise the egg.[39] Studies have shown contrasting results with supplementation, with some showing improvements in sperm concentration, motility and count, but others showing no improvements.

For women, zinc is important for egg growth and embryo development, and deficiency may prevent ovulation.[38] Although severe deficiency is rare, mild to moderate deficiency may be common and the WHO estimates that over 80% of pregnant women worldwide do not eat enough zinc. If the mother is low in zinc, the baby's levels may also be affected via the placenta. It is also linked to pre-term birth as a number of hormones important for the onset of labour are altered, and there is an increased risk of infections linked to premature birth. This is due to zinc's important role in strengthening the immune system. However, supplementation is not the answer as studies looking at this have shown conflicting results and there is insufficient evidence to recommend women take zinc supplements.[36]

It is very easy to meet zinc needs via the diet and the reason I do not recommend supplements is because excess may be damaging. Daily needs are 8 mg for women and 11 mg for men, and the Department of Health recommends that people do not exceed 25 mg of zinc in a day. There are supplements on the market that contain this high a dose, and these should certainly be avoided. The recommendation stands for a number of reasons:

- Excess zinc can cause gastric symptoms like nausea, abdominal pain, vomiting and diarrhoea.
- It can also result in headache and irritability.
- It may affect copper absorption, which can lead to iron deficiency and reduced immune function.
- It may also cause heart problems.

- It can affect the release of certain enzymes from your pancreas, which can mean that your body is unable to digest carbohydrates and proteins. This can then lead to diarrhoea, weight loss and malnutrition.

So, my overriding message here is that dietary sources are nearly always better than supplements and you will not overdose on zinc if you get it from your diet.

You can see the content of various zinc-containing foods in Table 5 but I would recommend that men try to get into the habit of including a variety of seeds, especially hemp, pumpkin, sunflower and sesame on a daily basis. These really are powerhouses of zinc, with 2 tbsp providing between 1.5 and 2.5 mg. Ground flax can also be a useful contributor but it does contain much less than the other seeds, with 2 tbsp providing around 0.6 mg. You can add seeds into your diet in a number of ways but here are some ideas:

- Sprinkle chia and sunflower seeds on your porridge for a bit of crunch.
- Add pumpkin seeds on top of sweet potato mash.
- Sprinkle them over a pasta dish for a lovely texture combination.
- Add sesame seeds to your stir fry, which also gives a great dose of calcium.
- Try sprouting seeds as this increases the availability of zinc for absorption (see below).

To ensure adequate intakes of zinc, aim to eat all the macronutrients with every meal, so that means a good source of carbohydrate, protein and fat. This could look like a bowl of porridge with almond butter stirred through and topped with mixed seeds and berries, or toast with nut butter and banana. For lunch you could have a sandwich with hummus, avocado and salad, and for dinner quinoa with beans, mixed vegetables and a cashew sauce. Throw in some dark chocolate as a snack and you have comfortably met your zinc requirements if you are a man, and slightly exceeded them if you are a woman.

Zinc absorption

It is good to be aware that zinc absorption is reduced in the presence of phytates, which are found in foods like whole grains, cereals and legumes. There are ways around this though:

Soaking: If you are using dried beans, lentils or chickpeas, put them in a bowl, cover with water and let them soak for at least two hours, preferably overnight. This increases the availability of the zinc, along with the other minerals such as iron, so you absorb them better. You can also do this with seeds, nuts and grains.

Sprouting: You can take your soaking a step further and start sprouting. This is actually really easy to do and there are lots of videos online, but you just need to follow a few basic steps:

- After soaking, put whatever you would like to sprout in a jar but don't fill it too much or it will get overcrowded once the sprouting starts. You only need to fill around a quarter of the jar. You also don't need any special sprouting equipment which can be expensive, but worth the investment if you are going to do this regularly. Really all you need is a sterilised jar (put it through the dishwasher first) and something with little holes in it to cover, like a cheese cloth.
- Leave the jar at an angle so any excess water drains out and leave somewhere out of direct sunlight as if it gets too warm your sprouts will go mouldy. (I know this from personal experience!) Then all you need to do is rinse your sprouts twice a day, with the lid on, draining any excess water each time.
- You will know when you have been successful as you will see little tails developing – it's really fun to watch these

grow. Once they are fully sprouted, pop them in a sealed container in the fridge and use within two days.

NB: Always smell your sprouts before using them. You will know when they have gone off as they will smell awful. Never use them if you are unsure and if you have a weakened immune system or if there is a chance you could be pregnant, do not eat raw sprouts as there is the potential to introduce salmonella, listeria or E. coli, all of which can make you very ill and harm your developing baby. If you cook them well that is absolutely fine and they will provide a very nutritious part of your meal.

Iodine

Iodine is a trace element on a par with folic acid (page 137) and choline (page 166) in terms of its importance for the health of the developing foetus. It also plays a key part in male and female fertility.

Iodine is an essential nutrient for thyroid health. The thyroid is a gland in the front part of your neck and is commonly known as the butterfly gland because of its shape. Thyroid function is regulated primarily by thyroid stimulating hormone (TSH), and its secretion stimulates the thyroid to take in more iodine from the bloodstream. This enables the thyroid hormones T3 and T4 to be made and released. If you do not have sufficient iodine stores, TSH levels remain high and the thyroid becomes swollen in its attempt to trap more iodine to enable it to make its hormones.

In terms of the health of the developing foetus, adequate iodine supply to the thyroid is essential as its hormones play a key role in brain and nervous system development. If the mother does not have sufficient iodine intake, there is an increased risk of intellectual impairment, with the most severe form being 'cretinism', and also infant death. Iodine is so important for the health of the child that it is classed as a key nutrient for the first 1000 days of life – that is, from conception until just before the child's second birthday.

For female fertility, a recent study found that moderate to severe iodine deficiency in urine samples of 501 women trying to conceive without a history of subfertility resulted in them taking significantly longer to fall pregnant.[41] There was a 46% reduced chance of becoming pregnant each cycle compared with women who had sufficient levels of iodine in their urine. Women who had mild deficiency had a small increased time to pregnancy, but this wasn't significant, suggesting only a modest risk, if any. Worryingly, over half of the women in the study had some level of iodine deficiency, with almost a quarter in the moderate to severe range. There were some limitations to the study, including the mainly white study population, and their urine only being tested at the start of the study so their levels may have varied after that time. However, it still remains a useful study in showing the potential effects of iodine deficiency on time to pregnancy and the importance of ensuring adequate iodine intakes for fertility.

Although severe iodine deficiency is very rare in the UK, mild to moderate deficiency appears to be a concern for women of child-bearing age and in pregnancy. The significant effects on thyroid hormones of low iodine status can impact a woman's menstrual cycle, making it more difficult to conceive, so it is really important to ensure adequate intakes. Recommendations for iodine intake in the UK differ slightly, with the Department of Health recommending 140 mcg a day, while the British Dietetic Association recommends intakes of 150 mcg daily for adults, but this increases during pregnancy to 200 mcg a day. This is to account for the surge in thyroid hormones during early pregnancy, possible increased losses in urine, and also to ensure the foetus gets enough to be able to make its own thyroid hormones once its thyroid gland has developed after around week 18 of pregnancy.

We need to get the right balance of iodine as too much can also have negative health implications. The foetus' thyroid is vulnerable to excess iodine and excess can increase the risk of their being born with thyroid disease. It can also have the same effect on our health as adults, with prolonged high doses causing disruptions in hormone production. For men, excess iodine intakes have been associated with reduced sperm motility, lower sperm counts and longer time to pregnancy. Lower sperm count and concentration have been found in men who are either deficient in iodine or taking in excess.[42] Men with optimum iodine intakes have been shown to have improved sperm parameters, with the role of iodine in enabling the thyroid to produce sex hormones being a likely mechanism. One of those sex hormones, testosterone, is involved in the making of new sperm and in sperm count, motility and structure, so having good circulating levels is important.

So how can you make sure you are meeting your iodine needs on a plant-based diet? Well, the only consistent way to do this is to take an iodine supplement in the same way as you would B12. Again, theoretically you can meet your needs by regularly consuming certain seaweeds, specifically nori and dulse flakes. However, seaweeds can contain varying amounts of iodine and it would be very easy to have too much, so regularly eating seaweed is not recommended, especially during pregnancy. In particular, you need to avoid kelp, and that includes kelp-derived supplements. This is because kelp can contain huge amounts of iodine and for this reason it is not recommended in any dose. You don't need to worry though if you enjoy eating nori and/or dulse flakes as they are fine to include in your diet from time-to-time, just not every day. For reference, one 2 g sheet of nori contains roughly 42 mcg of iodine, but the equivalent 2 g of dulse contains around 150 mcg. Dried wakame is also high in iodine, with 2 g providing 344 mcg. To give you an idea of how much iodine kelp can contain, just 2 g of dried kelp may contain a massive 2654 mcg![43]

It's worth mentioning that if you enjoy a side of crispy 'seaweed' when out for a Chinese, you don't need to worry about the iodine content. It doesn't actually contain any seaweed at all; it is made from spring greens.

For women trying to conceive, taking a 150 mcg supplement daily will be sufficient, but during pregnancy additional thought is needed. The easiest way to meet your needs without relying on regular seaweed is to drink fortified plant milk, aiming for 400 ml daily. This has the added benefit of helping you meet your calcium needs, particularly if you have higher needs than the general population. If you think about how to make this a part of your daily diet, it is pretty straightforward. You can make your oats with it or pour it over breakfast cereal, have it in your cups of tea (if you are a tea lover like me you could easily get through 200 ml in a day), or make a smoothie. You can also use it to make a cashew sauce for your pasta, black bean pancakes (see recipe below), or to make custard.

Black bean pancakes

- 140 g oats
- 230 ml oat/soya milk
- ½ tin black beans, drained and rinsed
- 1 small carrot, peeled and grated
- 1 tbsp chia seeds
- 1 small banana

Method
1. Put all the ingredients in a high-speed blender and blend until smooth.
2. Using a non-stick pan, spray on a little oil and cook three pancakes at a time.

3. Have as a snack on their own or with nut butter.
4. They freeze well so can be made in batches and kept when you need a handy grab-and-go snack.

Iron

Haem vs non-haem: what is the difference?

Haem iron is the iron found in animal products and you may have heard it said many times that you need to eat red meat in order to prevent iron-deficiency anaemia (IDA). This is so far from the truth. IDA is the most common nutritional deficiency in the world among any dietary patterns, including those that involve meat. It is certainly not specific to those following a plant-based diet.

There is also the argument that haem iron is better absorbed by the body. While this is undeniably true, actually it may not be a good thing. The problem is that it is too readily absorbed and once this happens, the body has a limited ability to get rid of it again. As haem iron is a source of oxidative stress and can cause damage to cells and DNA, this isn't a good thing. Non-haem iron, on the other hand, which we get from plants, is much better regulated by our bodies. Our absorption increases when our stores are low, and decreases when stores are plentiful. This clever regulation by our body may be its way of telling us that it wants iron from plants!

In terms of fertility, diets higher in haem iron are associated with higher rates of ovulatory infertility in women, while diets higher in plant protein and non-haem iron are associated with lower rates.[19]

In men, consuming iron in either low or high amounts may compromise fertility as it can interfere in the making of sperm, negatively affect libido and result in oxidative stress in the testicles and sperm.[44] The reason that iron deficiency can have significant effects on sperm quality is down to the fact that the making of sperm requires a lot of oxygen. When IDA is present, testicular blood oxygen levels are relatively low. This means the testicles are not able to increase total blood flow and sperm quality is reduced. IDA may also be triggered by inadequate dietary **copper**, and deficiency in this mineral is also associated with reduced male fertility and a reduction in libido.[44] It is therefore important to make sure you are also eating enough foods that contain this mineral also and there are plenty. They include whole grains, nuts, seeds, avocados, cucumbers, dried fruit, kiwis, mangoes, peas and potatoes. Just having one serving (30 g) of cashews, or pumpkin/sunflower/sesame seeds, will mean you consume sufficient amounts of copper. As with iron, too much copper can also cause damage to cells and DNA, and for this reason supplements should be avoided.

Iron absorption

There are some important things to consider when eating meals and snacks containing non-haem iron as certain nutrients can help you absorb it better and certain nutrients and components of foods can stop you from absorbing it very well. The most important nutrients to have with every meal and snack to help you absorb iron efficiently are vitamin C and carotenoids, and if you are eating a plant-predominant diet this will not be difficult to achieve. All you need to do is include vegetables or fruit, so if you are having peanut butter on toast, just put some blueberries on top or add them on the side. If you are having a portion of nuts then include some apple slices or a satsuma as well. With your main meals, always have at least two portions of vegetables and top your breakfast cereal or oats with berries or fruit of your choice.

Things that interfere with iron absorption are the polyphenols found in tea, coffee and red wine, and phytates and oxalates in some foods. Cocoa and calcium also reduce absorption. There are lots of ways around this though. Always avoid tea or coffee with your meals, and I would say leave at least 60 minutes either side. This can be tricky at breakfast if you are used to having caffeine when you get up and I can totally relate because initially I found it difficult to break that habit. What I would advise is, if you can't cope without your morning tea or coffee, have that first, go and have a shower and get ready and then have your breakfast. Even waiting 30 minutes can mean you will absorb more iron from that meal. With oxalates in some leafy vegetables, such as spinach and Swiss chard, these can be reduced significantly by boiling and less so by steaming. Phytates can be reduced by soaking legumes, nuts, seeds and grains and by sprouting. I wouldn't get too concerned about the calcium in plant milks at breakfast, as long as you are getting that vitamin C in. The main concern is if you are on calcium tablets which contain much more calcium in one tablet than you would get from your plant milk. Just take them two hours either side of a meal or snack and you will be fine.

Choline

Choline is a nutrient that may be found in higher quantities in animal products but can also be found in numerous plant foods. It is more commonly known to be essential during pregnancy as, like folate, it can also help to reduce the risk of neural tube defects (NTDs), but it is also important for fertility. In men, low intakes are associated with reduced sperm motility.[29] In women, there is little evidence relating to the preconception period but as it is so vital in pregnancy it is important for all women trying to conceive to ensure they are having adequate choline intakes. During pregnancy, choline requirements increase to support the growth and development of both the placenta and the baby, especially during the third trimester.[45] Many women prefer to take a choline supplement during the preconception phase and this is very much a personal choice and one I support, but I do not routinely recommend a supplement as it is possible to get all the choline you need from your diet. You can use Table 5 (see page 143) to check how much choline is in common foods in a plant-based diet and aim to eat these on a regular basis. Some plant-based eaters still include eggs in their diets and, if this is the case, you will get about 147 mg per egg.[46]

Calcium

Calcium is the most abundant mineral in the body, with 99% found in teeth and bone. In addition to several other nutrients including vitamin D, magnesium and phosphorus, it is essential for the contraction and relaxation of muscle, including the heart. It also enables blood to clot normally, and helps build and maintain strong bones. For the general population, 700 mg a day is adequate but for some groups this is set higher at a minimum of 1000 mg. This includes those with inflammatory bowel disease and coeliac disease due to the risks of malabsorption, and post-menopausal women who do not have the bone protective effects of oestrogen.

For male fertility, calcium has an important role. It regulates sperm motility and is involved in enabling effective fertilisation. Semen actually contains two to three times greater amounts of calcium than the blood, suggesting it has an important role in sperm development and function.

Calcium also appears to play a part in female fertility, especially during the development of the egg.[49] It is also important during pregnancy, although requirements do not increase until breast-feeding. During this time your needs are 1250 mg daily, so it is essential to re-evaluate your calcium intakes and ensure you are meeting these increased needs.

Many critics of plant-based diets will tell you it is not possible to get enough calcium without having dairy but this is nonsense; it is actually very easy. It is important though to be aware of individual needs and how to meet them. There is also evidence that dairy is protective against colorectal (bowel) cancer, but when you look at what it is that offers that protection, it is likely the calcium, an important fact that is often overlooked. The exact mechanism behind why calcium is protective is not clear, but we do know that calcium binds with fatty acids and bile acids in the gut to reduce their ability to damage cells in the lining of the large intestine. This damage, if it takes place, prompts the cells to multiply to try and repair the damage. It is during this rapid change process where the risk of abnormal cancer cells developing occurs. There is also evidence that dairy is linked to an increased risk of other cancers, including prostate[50] and breast cancer, and for this reason the World Cancer Research Fund do not make any recommendations for dairy intakes.

How can you ensure you are eating enough calcium?

Fortified plant-based milks and yoghurts are a really simple way to add to your daily calcium total as per 100 ml they contain exactly the same amount of calcium as the dairy alternative. Having just 400 ml a day will provide almost 500 mg of calcium. Avoiding for-tified products and choosing organic versions make meeting your calcium needs much harder and I always try to encourage my patients to switch back to the fortified versions if they are relying on organic brands. This is often a result of concerns over the addi-tives in these milks and/or misinformation, especially around soya milk where concerns are that non-organic brands use genetically modified (GM) soya. While it is true that most soya is genetically modified worldwide, and used in animal feed, this is not true for all soya used for human consumption. If you look at individual web-sites, they will tell you whether the soya used in their products is GM. Some also state it on their packaging, with one major non-or-ganic company stating clearly that they use ethically sourced, non

GM soya. With the additives, including gums and oils, yes there is some evidence that gums can have a negative impact on your gut environment, and added oils may not be ideal. The bottom line is though there is a much higher chance of long-term health problems if you do not get enough calcium, vitamin D and iodine, and most of these milks are an excellent source of all of these nutrients.

What is GM food?

If a food has been genetically modified, it means either a gene has been transferred from one living thing to another, or the genetic material, or DNA, has been altered in a way that does not occur naturally. There are many reasons for this, for example if a plant has been shown to be resistant to pests their genes can be transferred to another plant to also improve their resistance. Altering DNA can mean that a gene can be switched off to prevent something happening. For example, if a vegetable goes mouldy very quickly, the gene involved in this can be switched off making the vegetable last longer.

There are currently strict safety regulations in the UK under the Food Standard Agency (FSA) for all food products that have been GM. Foods must state on the label if any ingredients have been produced from genetically modified organisms (GMO). However, products from animals that have been fed GM animal feed do not have to be labelled. The safety assessments by the FSA include whether the food could be toxic or cause an allergic reaction. It will then only be authorised to be sold for human consumption if it does not pose a risk to health.

Another soya product, tofu, can be an excellent contributor to overall calcium intakes, with brands that are calcium-set being especially rich sources. For this you want to look for calcium sulphate in the ingredients and, in contrast to milks and yoghurts, organic versions are fine to choose as they are able to be set with calcium, although not all are, so always check the label.

Other useful sources include the majority of leafy green vegetables, with the only exceptions being spinach and Swiss chard because of their high oxalate content. Oxalates are naturally occurring compounds in plants that bind to calcium and other minerals in the body and reduce their absorption. However, as the oxalate content can be reduced by boiling the vegetables and these particular greens are really useful sources of a number of other very important nutrients, they should still be included in the diet. For reassurance, because I am asked this frequently, if you have another really good source of calcium on your plate alongside spinach, it will not prevent you from absorbing the calcium from the other food.

Nuts and seeds are also great sources of calcium, especially poppy, sesame and chia seeds, almonds and almond butter, beans, blackstrap molasses, and fruit including oranges, blackberries, pink grapefruit and dried figs. Table 6 gives a breakdown of foods and their calcium content.

Looking at Table 6, you can see how easy it is to meet even higher calcium needs. If we use the example of a female with Crohn's disease who will need a minimum of 1000 mg daily: if she had 400 ml of fortified milk on her breakfast and in cups of tea during the day or in a smoothie, fruit with fortified yoghurt for a snack, chia seeds on her porridge/breakfast cereal, and a tofu stir fry for dinner, she would have consumed just over 1000 mg without any effort at all.

Table 6: Useful plant-based calcium contributors[48]

Food	Portion size	Calcium content (mg)
Calcium-set tofu	80 g	320
Fortified milk	100 ml	120
Fortified yoghurt	100 g	120
Chia seeds	30 g	135
Poppy seeds	30 g	250
Sesame seeds	30 g	175
Tahini	30 g	43
Almonds	30 g	50
Almond nut butter	30 g	110
Edamame beans	100 g	45
Kidney beans	100 g	28
Chickpeas	100 g	38
Kale	100 g	40
Bok choy	100 g	68
Butternut squash	100 g	35
Wholewheat bread	2 slices	95
Dark chocolate (70-85%)	30 g	24
Black strap molasses	15 g	80-200

The wonder of herbs and spices

Herbs and spices are both fantastic foods to include daily in a plant-based diet, or indeed any dietary pattern, as they have a range of different properties that are beneficial to health and therefore to fertility.

The main difference between a herb and a spice is that herbs always come from the leaves of a plant whereas spices come from any part except the leaves. For example, cinnamon comes from the bark, ginger and turmeric from the root, and cloves and black pepper from the fruit or berries. Spices can be bought in their powdered form, as seeds, or as a whole root.

Herbs and spices are associated with many potential health benefits due to their anti-inflammatory, antioxidant, antimicrobial properties, and are protective against many chronic diseases. These benefits are largely a result of the actions of the phytochemicals they contain, especially polyphenols. The actions include positive effects on inflammatory pathways in the body and on the immune system.[51]

The main type of polyphenols found in herbs and spices are flavanols and flavones. These contain higher amounts per gram in comparison with other polyphenol-containing foods such as berries, allium vegetables (including onions and garlic), and dark chocolate. To give an example, 100 g of broccoli contains around 200 mg of total polyphenols, while turmeric has just over 2000.[52] This doesn't mean that in real terms turmeric will provide higher quantities because no one is going to eat 100 g of turmeric in one go. To convert into standard portion sizes, per teaspoon turmeric contains approximately 106 mg, and 80 g of broccoli contains approximately 160 mg. However, weight for weight herbs and spices are the winners.

Polyphenols and other compounds in plants are also known to exert antibacterial and antiviral properties and it is for this reason that they are often used as food preservatives. The essential oils found in certain herbs and spices, including cinnamon, thyme and oregano, have been shown to protect against some food-borne bacteria and fungi.[52]

A review looking at 25 different herbs and spices found that 84% had been found to have anti-inflammatory properties in at least one published study, with the most commonly studied varieties including thyme, oregano, rosemary, sage, basil, mint, dill, parsley, lemon grass, turmeric, cinnamon, clove, nutmeg, ginger, fenugreek, chili pepper, and black pepper.[51] Examples of anti-inflammatory compounds include curcumin in turmeric, gingerol in ginger and capsaicin in chili.

Consumption of herbs and spices differs throughout the world, with Europe being the lowest consumers at around 0.5 g per person per day. India, South Africa and Latin America are the highest consumers, averaging at 4.4 g per day, almost nine times higher than Europeans. In India, turmeric is the predominant spice, accounting for around 1.5 mg daily, 35% of total daily herb and spice intake.[52]

Cinnamon is one of my favourite spices and is an excellent choice to help manage blood glucose levels for those who are diabetic or women with PCOS who experience insulin resistance. Cinnamon can be used in a variety of ways: as a base spice in cooking, stirred through cooked porridge with some grated apple, added to a smoothie, or sprinkled on top of plain soya yoghurt or an alternative plant-based yoghurt with some fruit.

Herbs and spices are also excellent sources of a range of vitamins and minerals. Parsley, for example, contains high levels of vitamin K, as well as being a useful source of vitamins A and C, potassium, copper, calcium and magnesium. As you now know, the majority of these micronutrients have a role in male and female fertility, so pack those herbs and spices in!

Top tip: If you find that you buy herbs and then forget about them until they are beyond their best, try freezing them straight away. I have a drawer in my freezer dedicated to herbs and that way you can just pull out what you need, add it to your cooking and know that you will always have them to hand whenever you need them. Parsley and coriander don't even need chopping when you do that because you can just crumble them straight into your dish. I also keep some lemon slices in the same drawer in case I have forgotten to buy fresh lemons.

Spiced porridge

- 40 g oats
- ½ tsp each of cinnamon, ground ginger and turmeric
- 2 twists black pepper
- 150 ml plant milk
- Handful of berries
- ½ banana, sliced
- 5 walnut halves, crushed

Method
1. Put the oats in a small pan, along with the spices and pepper.
2. Add your plant-based milk of choice and simmer slowly until it is the desired consistency. (You may need to add a touch more milk.)
3. Serve topped with the fruit and walnuts.

14

Pillar 2: Exercise

Although I wouldn't go as far as to say that exercise is as important as diet in protecting yourself against chronic disease and optimising your fertility, they do go hand in hand. You cannot achieve optimum health if you eat well but don't exercise, or if you exercise regularly but eat a poor quality diet. So, in addition to forging positive eating habits, exercise is something that should always be incorporated regularly into your life because the benefits are plentiful.

I don't like the focus ever to be on weight because I believe that focusing on health is far more important psychologically when it comes to exercise. If you are exercising with the sole intention of losing weight, it can be harder to stick to your exercise regimen because it is easy to become demotivated and disillusioned. Exercise should be fun and it is important to find something that you enjoy. Some people love the structure of the gym and the classes offered, but this doesn't work for everyone and there is also a cost implication. Remember that any form of exercise that gets your heart rate up is going to be beneficial. It will improve your circulation, which will help to reduce the risk of heart disease and keep your sexual organs functioning. Exercise is also associated with improved mental health over time. It releases happy hormones so your daily mood can be improved too.

As with most things in life though, too much as well as too little exercise does have the potential to be harmful, and this applies to both men and women. It's probably easier if I talk about the effects on male and female fertility separately, so let's start off with the effects on female fertility.

Exercise and women's fertility

Studies have shown that exercise is beneficial to fertility when it results in weight loss in women carrying excess weight. However, if exercise becomes excessive and consistently results in more energy expended than energy taken in, it will result in a long-term energy deficit. This can lead to hormone disruption and subsequent negative effects on the menstrual cycle. Vigorous exercise leading up to IVF treatment has been shown to result in negative treatment outcomes. When more than 2200 women undergoing IVF were studied, those who did four hours or more of cardio exercise a week in the year before starting treatment had a 40% decrease in live birth rate. They also had a a higher risk of their IVF cycle being cancelled and a lower chance of implantation success. Moderate exercise however is associated with higher rates of fertility, independent of weight.[1]

When women ask me how much and what type of exercise they should be doing, I advise to always aim for daily movement. This means trying not to sit down for too long and walk whenever you can. Then keep specific exercise sessions short and effective. By that I mean, if you are used to running, instead of going out for hours and running until you feel depleted, try running for 20-30 minutes so you feel energised. Similarly, strength training is really important and will stand you in great stead for labour and delivery, but don't push yourself into lifting really heavy weights if you are not used to it. Lift so that you are putting some effort in and can feel it, but don't over-strain and keep these sessions to two or three times a week. It may be helpful initially to ask a qualified trainer to advise you on your technique because if you're new to weights it can be easy to get the technique wrong and you will then leave yourself open to injury. Finally, and this is an important one: if you are exercising regularly you should make sure you are eating enough. This is a common mistake, especially when someone is actively trying to lose weight, and it is one of the reasons I like to focus on health and the need to fuel your body. If you do regular strength training, this type of exercise builds muscle which means you will continue to use more energy when you are at rest. If you are not eating enough for your body to draw from, it will turn to other sources of energy and initially that will be your fat stores. The last thing you want to do is deplete your fat stores, as fat plays such a significant part in hormone health and fertility. Of course, it will be beneficial to lose excess fat stores, but this should be done sensibly over time and not rapidly. If you do not have excess fat to lose and are putting your body in a regular energy deficit, it will soon start to break down your muscle and that can lead to really significant effects on your health. Your immune system will be affected, and it will prevent you from reaching your training goals as your muscle will be reducing rather than building.

It is worth highlighting that women can feel particularly tired around the time of their period and for some women during the entire second half of their cycle, so choosing yoga, gentle stretches and walks can be really beneficial and will stop you from pushing your body into a place it doesn't want to be.

If you exercise regularly, or are starting to build up your exercise regimen, I would advise you always to make sure that you aim for three good meals a day and then include protein-rich, carbohydrate-containing snacks in between to fuel your increased activity. These could be something really simple like peanut butter and banana on toast, a handful of mixed nuts with chopped fruit, or my energising snack bars (see recipe on page 180). You don't need to increase your protein intake significantly if you are exercising a few times a week, so don't worry too much about that. As long as you are including good sources with every meal and snack you will be getting all you need.

Top tip: I'm not a fan of weighing scales but if you do find that weighing yourself helps to keep you on track, do be aware that if you start doing strength training which will build muscle over time, you are likely to see the numbers on the scales go up. This is because muscle is denser than fat, but gaining muscle is a good thing. Measuring your waist circumference can be far more beneficial because, as you get fitter, you will notice a reduction in this area which is far better psychologically than watching the scales and believing you are gaining weight. And beware of 'smart' scales that claim to be able to measure your body composition' – these can be inaccurate and there are many factors that can affect the results day to day. These include how hydrated you are, when you last ate, when you last exercised and where you are in your menstrual cycle. Try to focus instead on how great you feel on your new regimen rather than what the scales are telling you.

What about men?

As for women, taking regular, moderate amounts of exercise is beneficial and it has been shown that men who exercise at least three times a week for one hour have better sperm parameters than men who exercise more frequently and more intensely.[2] For example, long-distance runners have been shown to have clinical signs of reduced sperm quality, including sperm concentration, motility and shape, as well as lower total testosterone. Cycling for more than five hours a week has been shown to negatively affect sperm motility and concentration[1] and, although this seems like a lot of cycling, if you commute to work and back on a bike you can easily hit this level. One reason for this is the amount of heat generated that is concentrated on the testicles. Sperm do not like heat so if the scrotum is unable to move the testicles away from the body to cool down because it is squished onto a seat, the sperm are going to be affected by the frequent, prolonged heat. Regular cycling may also increase the risk of erectile dysfunction (ED), with explanations including reduced blood flow and pressure on the nerves of the penis from long periods of time on the saddle.

ED may also, in part, be caused by continuous high-intensity exercise due to the effects on the body. If a man continuously over-exercises, he may suffer disruptions to his hormones, will become fatigued and will be more likely to lose his libido and struggle to get and maintain an erection.

Exercise and oxidative stress

We've talked about the effects of oxidative stress on the body and fertility, and intensive exercise may increase levels in the body while also decreasing antioxidants. That means that not only is there more stress going on inside the body, but the antioxidants have less ability to help fight it. Not all studies have found that exercise increases oxidative stress but many have found it does to some degree.[3, 4] It is not really known whether that means we should be taking in more antioxidants to combat the effects, but it is still sensible to eat plenty of foods that have antioxidant properties.

My advice for men is the same as for women. Moderate exercise is associated with a range of health benefits, including a reduced risk of cardiovascular disease, and therefore a reduced risk of ED. However, intense exercise may trigger the onset of ED and also create hormone disruption. If you are experiencing these symptoms and are feeling exhausted by your exercise regimen rather than energised, it is definitely worth reassessing and aiming to reduce the intensity. Listen to your body and if you feel that you are too tired to work out, just have a rest day or go for a gentle walk.

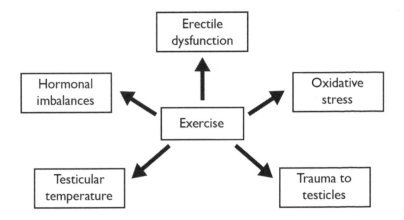

Figure 10: Potential ways in which exercise may affect male fertility

Remember, regular, moderate-intensity exercise is far more beneficial to all health outcomes than pushing your body into depletion.

Energising snack bars

- 180 g oats
- 2 ripe bananas (the more brown spots the better!)
- 1 tsp cinnamon
- 1 tsp ground ginger
- 2 tsp mixed seeds (pumpkin, sunflower, sesame, chia, linseed)
- 50 g ground almonds
- 50 g pecans, chopped
- 40 g dark choc chips (or a block chopped up)
- 25 g sultanas
- 75 g sweet potato, cooked

Method
1. Preheat oven to 180°C (350°F).
2. Chop the sweet potato up into small cubes and boil for 10 minutes, then mash well.
3. Mash the bananas in a large bowl.
4. Add the remaining ingredients and mix well until combined.
5. Press into a lined brownie tin or baking tray.
6. Bake in the oven for 25 minutes.
7. Cut into 9 larger squares or 12 smaller ones.

15

Pillar 3: Stress

Stress can be defined as 'any noxious event or episode which has the potential to be received as threatening, risky or harmful.'[1]

Stress is a bit of a complicated one because not all stress is bad for us. There are two types of stress: acute and chronic.

Acute stress can have some benefits. If you have a deadline, for example, the stress of that impending deadline can increase your concentration and productivity. If you have a deadline that is weeks or even months away, you might forget about that piece of work and focus on other things, but when that deadline starts to loom your focus might immediately sharpen and you will get it done. Acute stress can also be helpful in potentially risky situations. It isn't called your fight-or-flight response for nothing. Your senses become sharpened, your body releases hormones that result in increases in heart rate, breathing rate and blood pressure, and your blood moves quickly to your large muscle to prepare your body to fight or run away. Acute stress can vary significantly from your alarm clock waking you up in the morning to a physical danger. It is short-lived and usually passes quickly, but there are situations where it can turn into chronic stress.

One example of acute stress becoming chronic would be the stress you feel before a public speaking event. If you are uncomfortable in these situations, you will likely feel anxious and stressed leading up to it but this will pass once you have spoken and can relax. However, if public speaking is a part of your job and you are frequently feeling anxious and stressed, this can develop into chronic stress and is something that needs to be addressed.

I cannot emphasise enough how significant an effect chronic stress can have on your health. I would go so far as to say that it is at a level playing field with nutrition and, if it isn't addressed, quite simply you will not improve your health.

Your body's response to stress is instant and starts in your brain. It begins a series of interactions between the hypothalamus, pituitary and adrenal glands. This results in the release of adrenaline and cortisol, two of the 'stress hormones', from the adrenal glands. Once the stress has passed, your cortisol and adrenaline levels reduce back down. This step is really important as the communication between the glands in your brain and the adrenal glands on your kidneys also influences the production of sex hormones. If the stress doesn't pass, the stress response doesn't stop and this results in disruptions to your reproductive hormones. It is because of this that chronic stress may lead to poorer sperm quality and infertility in both men and women.

So, the effects of chronic stress on general health but also on fertility can be significant, and sometimes it feels like a bit of a vicious circle. Struggling to conceive is stressful, going through fertility treatment is stressful, and worrying about the effects of stress is stressful! Add that to general life stressors like work, relationships, social pressures, financial strains etc, and you can see how present stress is daily, even if you are not always aware of it. This is when the effects of such stress can start to become apparent in your state of health and affect your fertility, and this is why it is so important for both your mental and physical wellbeing to have in place some great stress management techniques.

In terms of fertility treatment, data show that men report feeling stressed providing sperm samples on the day of egg retrieval, and this may negatively affect overall semen quality, with effects on sperm concentration and motility. However, it is difficult to say whether stress results in reduced semen quality, or whether it is a consequence of decreased semen quality. Being diagnosed with infertility, frequent medical appointment, and failed IVF treatment are all very stressful events. It isn't just the stress itself though that can affect sperm quality; how you respond to stress may also play a part. Responding by being assertive or confrontational may negatively affect fertility by increasing adrenaline production which then results in the blood vessels in the testicles tightening. This reduces testosterone production and the making of new sperm,[2] so for men, stress management techniques are just as important as for women.

As stress causes an increase in cortisol and subsequent suppression of sex hormones, this can lead to a decreased sex drive and can also lead to undesired weight gain. Whereas acute stress is more likely to result in a reduced appetite, chronic stress is more likely to decrease behavioural control and increases impulsive behaviour. An estimated 35-40% of those experiencing stress increase their food intake.[1] The types of food likely to be chosen are foods high in sugar and/or fat, with low-energy, high-nutrient foods, particularly fruit and vegetables, decreasing. This may then lead to overeating, which in turn can lead to weight gain and potentially increase feelings of anxiety and depression. Conversely, some experiencing chronic stress may decrease their food intake, leading to weight loss, with potential adverse effects on their mood, energy, concentration and, for women, their menstrual cycle.[1]

Managing stress

In terms of stress management techniques, everyone is different, and what might work for one person may not necessarily work for the next. For example, I've had patients telling me that meditation is their idea of 'hell', but then when I explore further, I find their concept of meditation is sitting on a yoga mat, cross legged, with both hands raised, fingers touching, while gently humming. This stereotypical image does not reflect the broad spectrum of meditation and is very different to most people's practice.

If, like me, you find it difficult to still your mind and stop thoughts from racing in (I'm the same when I have a massage; I start thinking about all sorts!), guided mediation may be for you. Let me first explain some of the benefits of meditation:

- It can reduce anxiety and stress, and it can also help you respond to stress better and improve coping skills.
- It can lead to improved self-image and confidence: One meditation you can do is positive affirmations, where you repeat positive body image quotes out loud (I would recommend you do this one in the privacy of your own home!). Have you ever counted the number of negative things you say about yourself each day? I bet if you did you would be shocked. Can you imagine saying to your friends what you say to yourself? Repeating positive affirmations can really help switch the negativity off and lead to increased positive thoughts towards yourself and others. This can instantly improve your stress and anxiety. Your body is amazing; it is so resilient and it's yours. It is so easy to compare yourself with others but this makes you unable to appreciate what you have. Focus on all the incredible things your body can do and all the incredible things it is going to do from today onwards.
- It can improve your attention span: In this fast-paced world, we tend to flit from task to task and I really do think it can affect your ability to concentrate. Sitting and just allowing yourself to be still can enable you to improve your concentration and memory because your brain is focusing on just one thing rather than trying to keep up with multitasking.

The beauty of meditation is you can fit it in whenever you have a spare 15 minutes during the day, or even just five minutes. You may prefer to practise meditation before you get out of bed in the morning, or it may work better for you to take time out in the middle of the day, or before you go to bed. There is no right or wrong time, you just need to make sure you sit or lie somewhere comfortable, without being disturbed. You can then choose whatever form of meditation suits you on that particular day. You may feel you need to be energised, or you may need to unwind. You might fancy giving yourself a self-confidence boost, or you may need to clear negative thoughts. Whatever your need for that day, there is a form of meditation to suit it. Using guided meditations means your mind is less likely to wander because you are focusing on what the person is saying. Have a look online, or there are some great apps you can download onto your phone. It really is a wonderful practice and you will find, the more you do it, the more you will crave that daily time-out. Just make sure if there is anyone else in the house that you give them strict instructions not to disturb you. There's nothing less relaxing than someone bursting in half way through a meditation to have a chat (yes hubby, I am talking to you!).

Controlled breathing

Controlled breathing is another great stress management technique to master, and you can literally do it anywhere: on a train, in a lift, while stuck at traffic lights, before public speaking; any time you feel a little anxious and need to calm down.

There is no hard and set rule for controlled breathing. The only thing you need to remember is the outward breath needs to be slightly longer than the inward breath. So just experiment with what works for you in terms of time.

My favourite method is to inhale through my nose for four seconds, hold for two seconds and then exhale slowly out of my mouth for six seconds. Then you just repeat until you feel calm. No one needs to know what you are doing, and if it is safe to do so you can close your eyes for heightened relaxation. This is also an excellent technique to use before meal times if you suffer with tummy problems because it takes away any stress you may be feeling that can trigger symptoms when you start eating. Once you feel calm, you can eat knowing you are putting that food into a calm environment rather than a churning one.

Positive visualisation

This is something I did a lot when I was going through IVF treatment and it really helped me to stay positive and reduce my anxiety. However, I appreciate that it will not be for everyone as some people may not want to try it because they feel it risks raising their hopes. This is completely understandable, but actually positive visualisation can help to reduce those feelings of hopelessness and instead give you a brighter outlook and energise you. You can view it as a sort of focused day dream, where instead of drifting off, you focus your mind on what you want the outcome to be, concentrating on every step.

To put this into a fertility context, if you are trying to conceive naturally you can visualise these steps in your head:

See your ovary releasing the egg, imagine it moving down your fallopian tubes and meeting your partner's sperm. See the union and the fertilisation of your egg. Then visualise your womb, see how inviting it is, how thick the lining, how welcoming it is to your embryo. See the embryo burrowing into your womb's lining, making its home.

If you are going through fertility treatment, here is what you can visualise:

> Welcome each injection as a positive step towards your goal. Imagine the effects of the medications: see your follicles maturing and producing eggs, see multiple, good quality eggs. Project forward and visualise your medical team taking those eggs and introducing them to the sperm. Imagine them meeting and the sperm penetrating your eggs, fertilising them. See the day of embryo transfer and visualise your embryo meeting your womb, burrowing in and finding its home. See yourself with your baby, imagine yourself playing with him or her on the floor.

I visualised all of the above during treatment. My husband did not want to try it because he remained very emotionally detached during treatment out of fear of getting his hopes up too much, but for me it helped me to drown out the negative thoughts and gave me a sense of calm. I was telling myself every day the treatment was going to be successful by mapping out the whole process in my mind. Again, I know this won't be for everyone, and I am certainly not saying that you can determine the outcome of your treatment by visualising it. I do feel though that by focusing on the positives and crowding out the negatives you are giving your body the best chance. There is power in positive thinking. If you feel this may help you then try starting off with something completely unrelated to your fertility journey. Maybe there is a job you really want, or you want to overcome a phobia, or you simply want to feel less anxious about the world; try it and see what happens. If you feel it is something that works for you, you can apply it to your next menstrual cycle or fertility treatment.

Laughter therapy

Now this may sound like I'm going to tell you to join a group of strangers, link arms and force yourself to laugh hysterically while stood in a circle. Don't worry, this is not what I mean by laughter therapy.

Laughter is a positive sensation and it is addictive. If you hear someone laughing, especially those amazing belly laughs only children can do, you want to laugh with them. It is pretty much impossible to feel sad when you are laughing, apart from those times when you laugh so hard you start to cry. Laughter actively reduces stress by decreasing levels of the stress hormones, cortisol and adrenaline, and increasing the endorphins, dopamine and serotonin, your 'feel good' chemical messengers.

Probably the most stressful time of the trying-to-conceive process is that two week wait between ovulation and testing, or between embryo transfer and testing. This is the time I recommend my patients try laughter therapy, especially after intercourse and immediately following embryo transfer. There was a study conducted among women going through IVF who had just had their transfer. Half of them were entertained by a clown, and half had no intervention (the control group). Of the women who were entertained, 36% became pregnant. In comparison, 20% of the control group had a successful outcome.[3] I'm not saying you need to be entertained by a clown; for some of you that might significantly increase your stress hormones rather than relax you! But finding something that makes you laugh may be beneficial.

For me, it was watching my favourite comedian on my phone on the way home from the clinic and then resting on the sofa for a couple of hours watching TV, alternating between that same comedian and a show that never fails to make me laugh. Although I was aware that my sole aim was to laugh, it didn't feel forced in any way as I was watching something I genuinely found funny. It also took my mind off what had just happened and made me feel as though my little embryo had just been transferred into a happy and positive environment.

Dos and Don'ts

I can't say that I didn't worry at all during that two week wait as I think some degree of anxiety is inevitable when you are pinning so much on something working, but every time I felt as though my anxiety was starting to get too high, I would apply some or all of these stress management techniques to bring it down.

Another thing I would highly recommend, if it is possible for you after embryo transfer, is to book those two weeks off work, or at least the first week. You want to remain as calm and stress-free as possible during that time, not having to deal with the commute if you are not working from home; work stress is something that you just don't need. Also, finding something to occupy your mind is crucial so you don't spend long periods trying to second-guess whether you are pregnant. That can be really counterproductive, and please, STEP AWAY FROM GOOGLE! It can be so tempting to search the internet for 'signs I am pregnant' or 'what does implantation feel like?' but this can raise stress levels and mean that you are obsessing over the slightest little sensation. Try and spend those two weeks doing lovely things with either your friends or your partner. Go out for relaxing meals, watch a film in the cinema, organise a pamper evening, do some crafting – anything that helps you to relax and distracts you from negative thoughts.

And remember, if none of these techniques are for you, there are many other forms of stress management that can be equally as effective. These can be going for a lovely walk, or a gentle run outdoors in nature, curling up with a cuppa and your favourite book, or having a lovely warm (not hot) bubble bath. As long as you take some time out, away from your phone and other screens, and just focus on being present, you will feel much better for it.

16

Pillar 4: Toxic substances

In this section I talk about various substances that definitely have or may have adverse effects on both male and female fertility. While it may seem obvious to avoid smoking and significantly reduce or better yet avoid alcohol when you are trying to conceive, and also for your general health, there are some substances that you may not have considered. I have subdivided this section into smoking and vaping, alcohol, caffeine, air pollution, microplastics and BPA.

Smoking

Although this may seem so obvious – after all, we have been aware of the risks of smoking to our health for decades – unfortunately there are those who continue to smoke when they are trying to conceive. Numbers have fallen over the years, but in 2020 just over 22% of the global population were still smoking,[1] which I found really shocking. Cigarette smoke contains more than 5000 chemicals,[2] many of which are toxic to both men and women's reproductive systems. In fact, smoking is the number one cause of lead and cadmium exposure, both of which are associated with an increased risk of male infertility. Smoking is also a major lifestyle habit that causes oxidative stress in our bodies.[3]

For male fertility, this oxidative stress negatively impacts sperm quality. Studies have observed that smoking reduces sperm concentration and motility, as well as increasing sperm DNA fragmentation.[4] One study looked at over 2500 men and found the degree of reduction in sperm quality was linked to how heavily they smoked.[3] Heavy smokers had a 19% lower average semen concentration, 29% lower total sperm count, and 13% lower motile sperm compared with non-smokers. Smokers have also been found to have lower levels of antioxidants in their semen, giving less protection to newly developed sperm.[5] This is why smokers have higher requirements for nutrients that have antioxidant capacities such as vitamin C.

And as smoking is a major risk factor for heart disease, it is also a risk factor for erectile dysfunction, and also sexual dysfunction in women.

Some of the possible effects of smoking on the female reproductive function include early ovarian aging, poor quality eggs, disrupted sex hormones due to disruptions to the endocrine system, a significantly increased risk of ectopic pregnancy, and a less receptive womb environment which then impacts implantation.[6]

The majority of studies looking at both natural fertility and fertility treatment outcomes have supported an increased risk of infertility in female smokers. An analysis of several studies reported an overall 60% increase in the risk of infertility for women who smoke.[6] Worryingly, a recent study has found that mothers who smoke during pregnancy give their non-smoking daughters the same odds of subfertility at adulthood as smokers who were not exposed to cigarette smoke in pregnancy. This was compared to non-smoking adults who were not exposed to cigarette smoke in pregnancy.[7] The same study also found an association between mothers who smoke while pregnant and reduced testicle size, some abnormal sperm parameters, alterations to reproductive hormones and smaller final heights in male offspring.[7]

For women undergoing fertility treatment, those who smoke have been shown to have less successful IVF cycles and higher rates of ectopic pregnancy. For implantation and pregnancy rates passive smoking has been found to be just as damaging as active smoking.[6]

Although a causative effect has not been established, that is to say it cannot be said with certainty that smoking causes infertility, it is worth noting that there is no study that establishes that smoking causes lung cancer. This is because it wouldn't be ethical to conduct a randomised controlled trial where people were split into two groups: a smoking group who were told to smoke and monitored for signs of lung cancer over the proceeding years, and a control non-smoking group who were also monitored for signs of the disease. Instead, we have observational studies. These are studies where the participants are observed, without any interventions, in order for the researcher to draw conclusions. The first observational studies to suggest a link between smoking and lung cancer found there was an increase in deaths from lung cancer in the UK from around 1925, 15 years after tobacco and cigarette smoking became more popular. Since that time, many observational studies have demonstrated an association between smoking and an increased risk of lung cancer and the majority of the population would agree with this. Certainly, most people these days would not contemplate starting to smoke in adulthood because of that very real risk. So, in the same way as I would advise you to stop smoking for your general health, I would strongly advise both men and women trying to conceive to stop smoking and to reduce exposure to second-hand smoke as much as possible.

Vaping

Vaping is considered a safer alternative to conventional cigarettes. However, although vapes do not contain tobacco they do contain other harmful substances that may have negative effects on hormone balance and the normal functioning of the reproductive system. Research in humans is scarce and, although we cannot translate findings from animal studies onto humans, the data we have from such studies is concerning. This data includes negative effects on sperm quality, the implantation process and also pregnancy.[8] For this reason I would strongly recommend if you do smoke and are trying to quit, it is unlikely to be beneficial for your fertility journey to switch to vaping. Please do seek the right support to help you to give up without taking up another habit that may be just as harmful to your egg or sperm quality, as well as the implantation process and the health of your future baby.

Cannabis and other recreational drugs

Although large, high quality studies are lacking in terms of the effects of cannabis use on male fertility, data suggest there may be significant, negative effects.[9] The reason for this is that males have receptors for this drug throughout their reproductive system, including in the Leydig cells and Sertoli cells, in the back of the pituitary gland in the brain (remember this is where LH and FSH are created and released), and also in the testes. This all means that cannabis use can have a negative effect on male fertility by disrupting hormones and directly affecting spermatogenesis and sperm quality, including DNA damage. These effects may occur in men who do not use cannabis regularly as well as chronic users, as reviewed data suggests they may continue for a period of time after cannabis is no longer being used.

In women, a review found that although data are conflicting regarding the results of cannabis use and fertility, there is evidence that the drug increases the risk of disruptions to the menstrual cycle and ovulatory infertility.[10]

Cocaine use has also been shown to have deleterious effects on sperm quality, with reductions in sperm count and motility.[9] It is well known that if mothers take cocaine and other recreational drugs during pregnancy, there can be serious effects on the developing foetus. However, data showing the effects on fertility are conflicting. This is because studies in this area have been poorly designed, including inaccuracies in reported use by the participants, lack of clarity regarding the frequency and quantity of cocaine used, and also confusion over how recently the women used cocaine in relation to trying to conceive.[10]

To date I do not know of any data on the effects of amphetamine use and ecstasy on reproductive function.

With regard to the quality of evidence around recreational drug use and male and female fertility, it is clear that more robust data are needed. However, what we do have suggests potentially significant negative effects for both sexes and I would strongly encourage anyone taking these drugs to stop and to seek help if further support is needed.

Alcohol

This may seem a familiar scenario. You have a stressful day in work, or you have one of those days when everything goes wrong and the first thing you want to do is open the fridge and pour yourself a cold glass of wine. It's not uncommon for patients to tell me they have been advised to do this by their healthcare professional following a medical diagnosis to help them relax.

Worryingly, a study conducted by Drinkaware in 2018 involving 6000 adults aged between 18 and 75 found that almost 60% coped with stresses of daily life by drinking.[11] Reasons given included drinking to feel happier, to have more confidence in social situations, to forget their problems, and/or to reduce feelings of depression or nervousness. The problem is that, while drinking may help to relieve stress in the short term, in the longer term it can increase feelings of stress and anxiety and make stress harder to deal with. This may in turn increase the amount someone is drinking to try and achieve the same effects.

One way that alcohol may affect fertility is its role in vitamin B12 absorption. As alcohol acts as an irritant to the stomach lining, it results in reduced acid production. For optimum B12 absorption, stomach acid is needed and if alcohol is consumed regularly, over time the risk of B12 deficiency increases, even with supplementation. Other ways in which alcohol can impact fertility include its role as a source of oxidative stress and its potential effects on hormone production. These include increases in oestrogen levels which can negatively impact FSH levels and ovulation.[12]

While we know that drinking during pregnancy can have harmful effects on the developing foetus, including foetal alcohol spectrum disorders, still birth and miscarriage, the effects on female fertility are less certain. This is largely due to studies classing alcohol in different ways, with some describing specific quantities, and others using 'low', 'medium' or 'high' intakes, making it difficult to quantify. However, although studies on the effects of alcohol on natural fertility outcomes are conflicting, we cannot just discount the studies that have shown detrimental outcomes. It has also been demonstrated that both low and high alcohol intakes, defined as one drink a day and up to five units a day respectively, can result in longer time to pregnancy, a 50% reduced chance of conceiving and a lower implantation rate.[12] This suggests you do not have to drink large quantities for there to be an effect.

One large study reported that alcohol intake of any quantity did not adversely affect fertility in women under 30 but significantly did so in women above that age.[6] As many women are now delaying conception until this time it seems sensible to minimise alcohol consumption or, better yet, avoid it completely while trying to conceive. This applies to men as well, as alcohol is a source of oxidative stress, meaning that it leads to damage to cells and their DNA. It makes sense then to avoid drinking while you are trying to conceive so that the maturing eggs and developing sperm are not damaged by its effects.

Data relating to the effects of alcohol consumption on fertility treatment outcomes are also conflicting but there are not a huge number of studies. One study looking at Danish women undergoing fertility treatment found no association between low to moderate alcohol intake and the chance of a clinical pregnancy and live birth.[13] However, other studies have found that alcohol consumption in the year before treatment is associated with fewer eggs retrieved, and women who abstained from alcohol prior to treatment had higher pregnancy successes than women who continued to drink up to starting treatment.[14] A dose-dependent negative effect has also been shown on the quality of the embryo after fertilisation, meaning the risk increased along with alcohol intake.[15]

In men, significant associations have been found between high alcohol consumption and effects on sperm parameters. The problem again though is the frequent differences in what are classed as moderate and high consumption. In some studies, high alcohol consumption is classed as having eight or more drinks a week,[16] whereas in others studies it is classed as having more than two drinks a day. [4] This means more than 14 drinks a week. Even the moderate drinkers in this study were classed as having up to two drinks a day, but depending on the type of drink consumed could easily exceed government guidelines of no more than 14 units a week. This is because units vary considerably depending on what the alcoholic drink is. One standard glass of gin and tonic contains one unit of alcohol, whereas a glass of wine or pint of beer can contain up to three units. This means having seven gin and tonics a week equates to seven units, but drinking seven pints of beer, or large glasses of wine, can mean 21 units, exceeding UK government guidelines, and falling into the high consumption category.

There are data showing that couples where the male regularly drinks more than 20 units a week take longer to conceive.[5] This may seem like a lot to those who are irregular drinkers but it is not uncommon for me to see male patients with alcohol intakes in this region, particularly those with jobs that involve socialising with clients outside of work or those who have active social lives involving alcohol where six bottles or more can be consumed in one night.

There also appear to be differences in the effects of alcohol depending on whether a man is experiencing primary or secondary infertility. Primary infertility is when he has not fathered a child after a year of trying; secondary infertility is when he has fathered a child previously but has not conceived after a year of trying for a second child.[16] Again, in this study, the classification of moderate drinking differed from studies where number of drinks was used as a marker. This study used number of units, with eight units a week classed as moderate drinking and anything over that classed as heavy drinking, despite the lower end of the higher range being within government guidelines. This to me is a much clearer definition as it leaves no room for doubt and also falls into what I would class as being a more accurate marker of moderate drinking. The study found that men with secondary infertility were more likely to experience lower sperm concentrations if they exceeded eight units of alcohol a week, compared with moderate drinkers or those who did not drink alcohol at all.

The bottom line? As studies have shown conflicting outcomes for even mild to moderate drinking's effects on male fertility, my advice for men is the same as it is for women. It is sensible to address any factors which may reduce the chances of a successful pregnancy, and also to ensure the sperm quality is optimised, and a good way to do this may be to avoid alcohol when trying to conceive.

An extra consideration if you are a male partner, of course, is as a show of solidarity to stop drinking if your partner chooses to. This may be especially relevant to your relationship if you have previously socialised together where alcohol was involved, or if you have fallen into the habit of having a drink together at home in the evenings. Abstaining together is a great way to support each other along your fertility journey and hopefully into pregnancy.

Caffeine

Caffeine is a stimulant found in a number of foods and drinks, including tea, coffee, soft drinks, chocolate and herbal teas containing green tea. For the general population it is recommended that you should not exceed 400 mg daily, the equivalent of four cups of instant coffee. In pregnancy, it is half that amount and if you buy coffee from a high street store, it may contain your daily limit in one single shot cup.

For fertility, there are limited data showing that caffeine may negatively affect sperm health and time to pregnancy, but these findings were associated with caffeine in soft drinks rather than that in tea, coffee and hot chocolate. This may mean that the negative effects were due to the other components found in soft drinks, such as sugar and artificial sweeteners. A review in 2017 found little to no association between caffeine/coffee intake and the ability to fall pregnant but there were not enough suitable studies included in the review for a firm conclusion.[17] They did find that coffee consumption significantly increased the risk of miscarriage during early pregnancy but they could not state with certainty whether this was due to the caffeine or other components of the coffee.

As many women do not know they are pregnant during the early weeks of pregnancy, I would advise you look at how much caffeine you are having a day and see how you can reduce it. You can use Table 7 (opposite) to make a rough estimate of how much you are having on a daily or weekly basis and then aim to stick within the World Health Organization (WHO) guidelines of no more than 200 mg per day. This is during pregnancy, but I also advise this for everyone actively trying to conceive in case you do not know you are pregnant in the very early stages.

Table 7: Caffeine content of common drinks and foods

Food/drink	Portion size	Caffeine content (mg)
Energy drink	1 can	80-300
Filter coffee	1 standard cup (200 ml)	140
Instant coffee	1 standard cup	100
Cup of tea	1 standard cup	75
Cola	1 can	32
Diet cola	1 can	42
Green tea	1 standard cup	30-35
Matcha tea	1 standard cup	70
Chocolate (not white)	28 g	9-12
Decaf coffee	1 standard cup	7
Decaf tea	1 standard cup	2-10

If you are looking to reduce your caffeine intake, there are so many lovely alternatives to caffeinated drinks. These include the obvious decaf teas and coffees, although do be aware that they still contain small amounts of caffeine. Although the majority of decaf teas contain very small amounts, the content does creep up the longer it is brewed. Other great choices are herbal teas, but be careful with green tea and Matcha as both contain caffeine. Caffeine-free herbal teas include peppermint, lemon and ginger, rooibos, chamomile, hibiscus, rosehip and echinacea. It is important to note that not all herbal teas are safe in pregnancy - for example, liquorice tea is not recommended. Chamomile may also help you to sleep when used as a bedtime drink. Other delicious options are turmeric lattes, for an extra antioxidant boost, and beetroot lattes, both of which are commonly available in most highstreet coffee chains, although you can of course make them yourself.

Air pollution

For decades it has been suspected that air pollution is linked to a number of adverse health outcomes, including respiratory diseases like lung cancer and childhood asthma. If you travel to major cities, you can feel the amount of pollution in the air, especially when walking along the main roads, sat at train stations and navigating the underground.

But what about fertility? Does air pollution have a negative effect? The answer appears to be yes.

A recent study assessed the risk of infertility in over 36,000 nurses when looking at the distance between their halls of residence and the main road.[18] Those who lived less than 200 metres away had an increased risk of infertility compared with those who lived further away.

A recent review of 11 studies looked at the effects of air pollution on women of childbearing age and women undergoing IVF treatment.[19] The air pollutants investigated were separated out into various groups, some of which are not necessary to discuss, so I will just explain the findings from the four most relevant: nitrogen dioxide (NO_2), sulphur dioxide (SO_2), carbon monoxide (CO) and PM10 and PM2.5.

NO_2: Exposure to higher amounts of NO_2 was associated with a lower live birth rate in women undergoing IVF, and in the general population, although studies showed conflicting results regarding fertility rate and exposure to NO_2. In terms of the risk of miscarriage, the rate was much higher in women exposed to NO_2 compared with those who were not.

CO: Exposure to CO was associated with an increased risk of miscarriage in the second and third trimester.

SO_2: There was no significant effect for women going through IVF on birth rate, number of retrieved oocytes or embryos transferred, but in the general population there was found to be an increased risk of miscarriage as exposure levels increased.

PM10 and PM2.5: These are two types of air pollution that are thought to affect people more than any other pollutant according to the WHO. The 'PM' refers to the particles in the air, and the numbers are the size of the particles. Studies on the general population have shown conflicting results, with some showing no effects on fertility and others showing a significant reduction when exposed to both sizes of particle. For women going through IVF there was no negative effect on live birth rate, number of oocytes retrieved, embryos transferred or embryo quality. However, there was an increased risk of poor pregnancy outcomes, with an increased risk of miscarriage for women exposed to higher levels of PM10. The same risk was found for those not needing to go through fertility treatment. For males there also appears to be a risk from exposure to these particles, with negative effects on sperm shape and motility, as well as an increased risk of chromosomal abnormalities. This means changes to the number and/or structure of chromosomes that can lead to birth defects. Exposure to very high levels of air pollution has also been associated with damage to sperm DNA.

There are a number of potential reasons why air pollution can negatively affect reproductive outcomes. These include the possibility of them mimicking sex hormones and disrupting their actions in the body, and the promotion of oxidative stress and inflammation in the body.

We have to take the findings from this review[23] with a pinch of salt because there were several limitations and it's important to explain these. The reference level of each pollutant did vary between studies so more consistent data are needed. The population groups studied and the definitions used to assess infertility and miscarriage were also different, which means it is difficult to draw a general conclusion. As always, further research is needed, but the results of this review do seem to indicate an association between infertility, poor pregnancy outcomes and exposure to air pollution.

So, what can we do about it? While it is impossible to avoid air pollution completely in our daily lives, we can reduce our exposure by putting into place some simple changes to our daily routines.

- Consider altering your route. If you enjoy walking or cycling to work, or you just going for a daily walk or run, look at your route. Do you tend to stick to busy main roads? If so, see if it is possible to safely make any changes. I'm certainly not advising you to walk through an unlit park on your own or do anything that will compromise your safety – just do a bit of research and see if there is a less polluted route you can follow where you are not isolated.

- When driving, and especially when you are stuck in traffic, leave a gap between yourself and the car in front. This isn't just for general safety reasons; imagine all those fumes coming out of the exhaust of the car in front of you and heading straight through your vents. Leaving a larger gap reduces your exposure to those fumes.

- When you're stuck in a traffic jam, your exposure to pollution is much higher. The best thing you can do is close the windows and press the recycled air button. Doing this can reduce the amount of pollution inside your car by 20%.[20] This is compared to using the usual ventilation system that can expose you to up to 80% of the pollution outside your car. The only problem with using recycled air is if there are two or more people in the car with you; then it can get uncomfortable so it is advised to allow outside air in for one minute every 10 or 15 minutes.

- If you tend to exercise mainly outdoors, try substituting some of those sessions with indoor workouts, either at home or in other ventilated spaces. This way, you can halve your weekly exposure to pollution while still keeping fit. Of course, being outside with nature is vital to help keep your mental health optimised so if you exercise in areas where exposure to pollutants is much lower you won't need to do this. If you exercise where you are constantly being exposed to air pollution you may like to make some changes.

Indoor pollution

It is also important to be aware of the potential for exposure to indoor pollutants such as those brought in from outside, household chemical-containing cleaning products, and mould/fungus that grows in moist/humid environments. It is not possible to eliminate every single indoor pollutant but you can significantly reduce your exposure by doing the following:

- Hoover frequently and always remove outdoor shoes before stepping on your indoor carpets/flooring.
- Where possible switch your chemical cleaning products to toxin-free varieties. You can find these in supermarkets and zero-waste shops, as well as in some independent stores, or you could try making your own cleaning products. There are many books on this topic and you can also find plenty of information online.
- Avoid using indoor air fresheners, scented candles and incense as they can contain toxic compounds and can also trigger allergies.

Ensuring you keep your rooms well ventilated and investing in a dehumidifier can reduce the risk of mould, but with the cost-of-living crisis and substantial energy bills, many people will not be able to run a dehumidifier or heat their homes sufficiently. Recent events in the news have highlighted the health effects of being exposed to mould, especially for those with compromised immune systems, allergies or existing respiratory conditions such as asthma. These are some ways you can try to reduce the risk without significantly adding to your energy bills:

- When cooking, use the extractor fan when possible to remove excess moisture.
- Avoid drying clothes on radiators or indoor racks as much as possible as this can create damp. If you know there is no rain in the forecast try to hang your clothes on an outside line. Even in the winter on a dry day this can be really effective, especially in a strong wind. You could use a heated clothes rack for short periods on days when you can't use your outdoor line – putting a bedsheet over the top will retain the heat and they will dry quicker so you will use less energy.
- If you have cupboards and drawers in your house that you rarely use, open them to give them an airing every now and then.
- Clean regularly with your non-toxic cleaning products to prevent a build-up of mould on surfaces.
- Avoid carpets in rooms where moisture build-up is likely such as bathrooms and basement rooms.
- Maintain gutters and drains to prevent leaks.
- If you have large areas of mould, do call in a professional to help eliminate the problem.
- Always see your doctor if you feel mould is causing any health concerns.

Microplastics and BPA

Sadly, the plastic waste on our planet is everywhere, with around 6,300,000,000 tons generated between 1950 and 2015.[21] Most of this ended up in landfills and the environment, and once discarded plastic enters the sea, the action of the sunlight, waves and wind breaks it down into tiny particles called microplastics. We have all seen the heartbreaking footage on nature programmes where aquatic animals have ingested plastic, or have died due to their beaks/mouths being bound by plastic rings, or have become tangled in plastic nets and drowned. But what about the effects on our reproductive health of ingesting microplastics found in fish and seafood?

Microplastics have been found in human stool, showing that they do make their way into our digestive systems, and a recent study with a small number of participants found microplastics in four out of six placentas (samples were taken following safe delivery), with both babies and mums affected.[22] This indicates that, once in the body, microplastics can reach all areas of placental tissue and suggests possible consequences for pregnancy and embryo development and health, although more research is needed to assess this.

Microplastics are also associated with decreased fertility in both men and women due to plastic's potential disruptive effects on hormones,[23] and it isn't just the microplastics themselves that are a cause for concern. They also act as carriers for other chemicals, including plastic additives and environmental pollutants.

Minimising or eliminating fish and sea food can reduce our exposure, but what about plastics that some of us use daily at home or when we are out? These include plastic drinks bottles and containers, especially those made with bisphenol A (BPA). BPA is a chemical that has been used as a component of plastic for over 60 years.[23] It is widely used in the food industry in long-life food and drink containers, as well as being present in other items such as sunglasses, mobile phones, cosmetics and even fridges. This means we can be exposed to it through our skin and by inhalation as well as via our diet. However, it has been labelled as a substance of very high concern by the European Chemicals Agency since 2017 due to its potential disruptive effects on hormones.

In mice/rat studies, BPA has been shown to result in a significant decrease in sperm counts, motility, shape and DNA quality, as well as reduced testosterone levels. In humans, there is a lack of controlled trials as it would not be ethical to purposely expose the male to something that may harm his fertility. However, there are studies that have looked at semen quality in the general population,[25, 27] with some finding that men who had the highest levels of BPA in their urine had lower sperm motility than men who had lower levels in their urine. Higher levels of urinary BPA have also been associated with lower sperm counts, concentration and vitality, as well as an increased risk of sperm DNA damage.[21]

In contrast, other studies, including one looking at 556 Danish men aged 18-20.[24] found no association between urine levels of BPA and sperm quality, although exposure might have been too low in some studies to determine possible effects.

Similarly, not all studies on female fertility have found BPA exposure to have negative effects. However, there is evidence that infertile women have higher levels of BPA in the blood than fertile women, and that higher levels of BPA in the urine are associated with poorer egg maturation in women undergoing fertility treatment. Significant associations have also been found in women who have PCOS between BPA and raised androgen concentrations.[25] There is also evidence that higher levels of BPA in the blood have been found in women who have experienced recurrent miscarriages and an association has been suggested between BPA levels and premature birth.[23]

Interestingly, soya consumption may protect against the potential adverse effects on reproductive health of BPA. A subgroup of 239 women from the EARTH study[26] provided urine samples to test BPA levels at various points during their IVF treatment and were asked to complete a detailed questionnaire before starting treatment. One section asked them to detail how often they consumed one or more of 15 different soya-based foods in the three months prior to treatment. These soya foods included tofu, tempeh, processed soya-based foods, soya beans, soya milk, yoghurt and cream and soya-based protein, bars and drinks. Almost three quarters (74%) of the women ate soya in some form. Interestingly, in the women who did not eat soya, higher levels of BPA in their urine were associated with lower implantation rates, and lower clinical pregnancies and live births. In the women who ate soya, these associations were not found, even with equally increased levels of BPA. This study was small and more research is needed using larger numbers of women, and including men too. However, the possibility of soya being protective against the adverse reproductive effects of BPA is yet another great reason to include it in your diet. After all, it would be impossible to reduce our exposure completely to BPA, even with great effort, so if some of the effects could be buffered by the humble soya bean, well that's a great incentive to up your intake.

Existing studies on humans have their limitations – for example, different exposure levels to BPA within some groups, and the need to consider other factors that may have an impact on sperm and egg health and overall fertility. However, there is sufficient evidence to recommend reducing your exposure to BPA and microplastics as much as possible. My top tips are shown in the box.

How to reduce your exposure to BPA and microplastics

- Invest in a reusable, non-plastic water bottle and cup for hot drinks. It has been shown that the average person drinking three cups of coffee a day using disposable cups ingests around 75,000 tiny microplastic particles. This is because when the hot liquid is poured into the cup, the thin layer of plastic used to coat the inside of the cups releases the particles into your drink.[27] This is likely to apply to any hot drink consumed from a disposable cup. Using your own also of course has positive effects on the environment.
- Avoid storing food in plastic containers, especially if the containers have been heated previously – for example, using old takeaway containers for batch cooking storage.
- Avoid heating plastic containers in the microwave. If you are having a shop-bought ready meal, or takeaway, transfer the contents onto your dish and then heat. If plastic is heated it speeds up degradation and harmful chemicals can be transferred onto your food along with the microplastics.
- Avoid using clingfilm. As well as being damaging to the environment, the chemicals contained in the plastic can be transferred onto your food, especially as cling film often has to be peeled off the food when used as a cover during heating. I love silicone lids – they are non-toxic and free of BPA, can cope with a large range of temperatures and also keep your food fresh because they create such a tight seal when the right size lid is used for your container.

17

Pillar 5: Sleep

You all know how you feel after a rubbish night's sleep, like a sub-functioning version of yourself, and unfortunately sleep deprivation is becoming more common. Around 20% of adults are now sleeping less than the recommended seven to nine hours a night.[1] This means that around one in five adults are chronically sleep deprived.

Sleep deprivation can occur sporadically – for example, many women find they experience disturbed sleep just before and during their period, or certain life changes can mean temporary disruptions to sleep. However, it can also be chronic, caused for example by shift working, having a job that involves a lot of travelling or communications with countries with different time zones, lifestyle, or actual insomnia. This means when you regularly have problems sleeping, including struggling to go to sleep, waking frequently in the night, waking early and then being unable to go back to sleep, and waking feeling fatigued rather than refreshed.

There are two main types of sleep: rapid eye movement (REM) sleep and non-REM. Non-REM sleep is itself divided into three substages and it is in stage three that deep, restorative sleep occurs. REM is your dream sleep and it is also during this stage that memories are consolidated. Brain activity during this stage is really high, which is why you can sometimes have really vivid, realistic dreams. This is the stage where you can dream someone close to you has done something awful and then feel cross with them when you wake up because it seems so real.

The effects of sleep deprivation

A recent review found that long periods of sleep deprivation may affect male reproductive hormone balance in the long term because sleep deprivation induces the stress response.[2] This means cortisol is released, which in turn reduces testosterone production. Interestingly though, the review noted that day time testosterone levels are only reduced if men suffer sleep deprivation in the second half of the night, which is heavier in REM sleep. If the sleep deprivation occurs in the first half of the night there are no effects on day time testosterone levels. This implies that the timing of sleep deprivation is relevant, but more studies are needed.

We know that oxidative stress has negative effects on all kinds of system in the body. Poor quality sleep has been shown to cause changes in the body that exert the same effect as oxidative stress, which can result in high levels of corticosteroids in the blood. These are steroid hormones, and high levels are associated with infertility in both men and women.[2]

In women, even short-term sleep deprivation in the follicular phase (the first half of the menstrual cycle) is associated with an increase in thyroid stimulating hormone (TSH). High levels of this hormone are associated with disruptions to the menstrual cycle and an increased risk of miscarriage.

Oestradiol levels have also been shown to be altered with sleep deprivation, with women who do not have regular sleeping habits having higher levels of the hormone compared to those who have regular sleeping habits. This is significant as oestradiol is the main form of oestrogen in women of reproductive age and it plays an important part both in ovulation and in growth of the follicles in the ovaries.[2] This means that implementing a regular sleeping pattern may benefit overall reproductive health.

One of the difficulties in assessing whether sleep deprivation has an effect on female fertility lies in the fact that the group of women most often studied are night-shift workers. Although findings from this group are applicable to many women, they cannot be applied to women who work during the daytime hours. For women who do work night shifts, associations have been made between disruptions to the usual sleep cycle and altered length of menstrual cycle, infertility and miscarriage.[3] Other studies have found no association between shift work and infertility but have noted a 20% increased time to pregnancy for women working more than 40 hours a week. These women were nurses so, although it was not specified whether these hours were during the day or night, it can be assumed that some night shift work was included.[4]

The bottom line with sleep is we don't have enough data at the moment to say to what degree it may affect fertility. However, there are associations between sleep deprivation and disruptions to levels of key reproductive hormones as well as other negative effects on the body which in turn can affect fertility. Sleep is vital for the normal functioning of the body and brain and chronic deprivation is associated with an increased risk of many disorders, including depression, anxiety, high blood pressure and heart disease.[2] Prioritising sleep then should be at the forefront of your mind, both for reproductive and for general health. The role of sleep in health is the reason that restorative sleep is one of the pillars of lifestyle medicine, but unfortunately it is something that is often overlooked during a health assessment. If you are really struggling and have tried all the tips in the box then do see your GP before trying any of the marketed supplements available. These may help you sleep in the short term, but it doesn't solve the problem of why you are struggling to sleep and it is possible to become reliant on these supplements. In addition, many of them can make you feel very groggy for some time after you wake up which means spending even more of your day feeling fatigued. Your doctor may decide to refer you for talking therapy, or even to a sleep clinic, and they will be able to do any necessary investigations to rule out other causes.

Of course, sometimes there are periods in your life when sleep is unavoidably disturbed. If you are struggling with secondary infertility, for example, you may have a young child who regularly wakes you. The purpose of this chapter is not to make you feel anxious about how disturbed your sleeping pattern is, which in turn may prevent you from getting a peaceful night. The point is to highlight the importance of trying to implement a regular sleep pattern whenever you can. Sleepless nights are an inevitable part of everyone's life at some point. The aim is overall to get that magic seven to nine hours as often as you can.

Five tips to help you get a better night's sleep

1. Try to establish a regular sleeping routine by going to bed at the same time and waking at the same time, even on weekends. In time you will find that your body clock automatically wakes you without the need for an alarm clock, meaning waking in time to your rhythm rather than to a loud noise.
2. Address any anxiety that may be stopping you from getting a restful night. In addition to seeing your doctor, if you are really struggling it can be helpful to write down your anxieties in a note book or journal that you can keep on your bedside table. That way, you are taking the anxieties from your head and putting them on paper, then you can close your book and trap them inside there.
3. Try not to look at any blue light at least an hour before you go to bed as this can really mess up your ability to sleep by affecting the production of melatonin. Leaving your phone/tablet etc downstairs and finding a good book to read instead will help your body to wind down and prepare

for sleep. If you use your phone as your morning alarm, I would strongly recommend getting a small alarm clock instead or even using a smart speaker. This means if you do wake in the night you won't be tempted to check your phone to see what time it is and expose yourself to blue light when your body is needing darkness.

4. Make sure your room isn't too hot. Your body drops its core temperature by about 2ºC to enable sleep and 18ºC (64ºF) is the optimum room temperature, according to the UK's National Sleep Foundation. This is pretty much impossible to do during the summer months but I always find a good fan combined with a pair of ear plugs helps. Filling a hot water bottle with cold water can also be a godsend.

5. Practising meditation at bedtime can be very effective as this can activate your parasympathetic nervous system which leaves you feeling relaxed.

18

Pillar 6: Relationships

Infertility is stressful. There is no question about that. If you are trying to conceive naturally it can feel as though you are caught up in a monthly cycle of expectation and disappointment, and if you are going through fertility treatment you have to cope not only with the fear that it will not work but also the crazy effects those hormone injections have on your body. Trust me when I say I turned into an emotional wreck. One moment I felt as though I could burst into song and cartwheel around the room (not literally as I am the world's worst cartwheeler and would probably have ended up breaking something) and the next minute I was a sobbing, snotty mess because I put too much milk in my tea. The whole process of trying to conceive is one huge emotional and physical rollercoaster and when you are feeling that way it is often those closest to you who experience the brunt of it. That may be your partner, parent(s) or close friends, but it is really important to keep telling yourself that they are your support system and all they are trying to do is be there for you, even if sometimes you just want to close the door on them and be by yourself.

Everyone deals with emotions differently. Take my husband. He is brilliant at solving problems and if I ever need to get my head straight and come up with a solution to something, he is the best person to go to. But sometimes, you don't want a solution; sometimes you just need to offload and vent, and this is really important to communicate. The well-worn phrase 'communication is key' could not be more accurate when you are struggling to conceive.

So often, partnerships suffer during the fertility journey, whether it is because one partner feels they are shouldering the blame for the failure to conceive, or because each other's communication styles are different which may make one partner feel unheard or unsupported, or because you have become so emotionally drained and disheartened by the whole process you just don't want to talk about it anymore. It's hard, and it can be made worse by other people's insensitive comments, even if they may not mean them to be.

Remember, you are a team, and whether you are in a couple or are going through the process on your own, you need your team around you. Talking about your fears and worries is so important and I wholeheartedly encourage you to do that whenever you feel you need to. Sometimes though, a change of topic and scenery can work wonders, not just for yourself but for your relationship. So, the box shows my top tips to help you strengthen those bonds and keep your relationships healthy and thriving during your fertility journey.

Top tips to support your relationships

1. Understand each other: People have different ways of dealing with emotional situations. One of you might like to talk about things straight away, but the other may prefer to disappear somewhere to get their head straight. Neither one is right or wrong and that is really vital to remember. There is nothing more frustrating than your partner going silent, or walking off when you want to talk about things, but if you are not on the same page it means you are both entering a conversation on uneven ground emotionally. Have a quick chat, acknowledge how each of you is feeling and then agree to sit down and talk later that day once you have both had time to process things. However, and I

stress this point, allocate a certain amount of time to talk things through but don't let it consume you because it can become very easy to dwell on things and reach a point where your key emotions become anger and resentment. To stop this from happening see point #2.

2. Spend some quality time together and ban all conversation about fertility: This is so important because struggling to conceive can take over your entire life. Remember the people you were before and enjoy each other's company. Rather than going to the cinema where you can't talk, or going out for dinner where talking can become too easy and before you know it you are back on all things fertility, try doing something different. Axe throwing is supposed to be a great experience, and it has the bonus of being a physical activity so you can vent your frustrations at the target rather than at the person you are with!

3. Have sex for fun, not to conceive: Everyone who is trying to conceive will attest to the fact that sex becomes a regimental activity. Current advice is to have sex frequently rather than trying to track when you are ovulating and calling your partner mid work meeting to get home and do his business, but I haven't spoken to a single couple who really enjoyed their sex life when they were struggling to conceive. I even know one lady who drove two hours to where her husband was staying for work because her ovulation kit gave her a smiley face! Remember the sexual attraction that brought you together in the first place and enjoy exploring each other without the end goal being to conceive.

4. Be there physically throughout the IVF process: Although the emotional connection is so important, so is being physically present during the appointments, scans and injections. If

you have a partner, ask them to be by your side during all of these things because, although most partners will want to be there during the hospital appointments, they may not feel the injections require their physical presence and may happily leave you to get on with them by yourself. Some women may be fine with that and may actually prefer it, but if you want your partner by your side while you do the injections, or even for them to do them for you, don't be afraid to tell them. It can create a new level of intimacy and bring you closer together, knowing you are doing everything you can together to help achieve what you both want most in the world. If you are going through the process alone, ask your mum or your friend to be by your side too. They may be there during the scans and check-ups but it can be a lonely process once you are home and I bet they will be delighted to be asked to share that experience with you.

5. Spoil each other: In a world where equality is key it is amazing how one sided this can be. Yes, it would be incredible to come home and your partner has run you a bubble bath, or they bring you a cup of tea when you wake up, or take over the dinner preparations for a night while handing you a specially prepared non-alcoholic cocktail and telling you to go and put your feet up. But, what about them? It is amazing how much small tokens are appreciated and how it really strengthens your bond and prevents the risk of one person feeling taken for granted. So, if you are guilty of being the one to take most of the time, try doing little things for them to show them how much you love them. It doesn't need to cost anything; a little note in their work bag, or a smiley blueberry face on their breakfast will do the trick.

> If you are the awesome person going through treatment single-handedly (and I seriously mean that), make sure you put time aside to pamper yourself. Book a lovely relaxing massage, or run a gorgeous bath with candles; anything that makes you feel rejuvenated.

All of the tips in the box can really help, but if you feel that your relationship is struggling, then please do not be afraid to get an outsider's perspective. Relationships can be fragile and if you have gone through several rounds of fertility treatment already, you may feel that you need that extra support.

Talking to your parents, work colleagues or friends can be really helpful, but they know you too well and can be too close to the situation. Plus, they will be fighting your corner and may well agree with you even if really they are thinking you could have done something differently. This means that any negative feelings towards your partner could unintentionally be fueled, which will not help your relationship. Speaking to a counsellor can really help because it both gives you both a safe space to voice your feelings and also helps identify things that may be causing conflict within your relationship that you have not been able to recognise on your own.

19

Common fertility nutrition myths

Seed cycling

'Seed cycling' is a popular approach to balancing hormones that can regularly be seen on social media and is often advised by wellness practitioners, but what exactly is it?

Advocates of seed cycling claim that consuming seeds during specific parts of the menstrual cycle can help regulate female hormones throughout the cycle.

They will tell you that during the follicular phase you should eat 1-2 tbsp of pumpkin seeds and flax seeds daily for the duration of the phase as they contain phytoestrogens such as lignans that can balance oestrogen levels. During the luteal phase, the types of seeds consumed change to support optimal progesterone production, and these include 1-2 tbsp of sesame seeds and sunflower seeds daily. As well as the phytoestrogens, advocates claim the zinc, selenium and vitamin E content in seeds also play a role in helping to balance hormones, and some will even claim these seeds need to be bought in their whole form and then ground before eating.

So, what does the science say?

Well, there are several reasons why a woman will experience hormonal imbalances and these include the hormone-driven conditions, PCOS and endometriosis, over-exercising, a thyroid disorder, or being over/underweight. For the general population with a healthy menstrual cycle, disruptions to reproductive hormone production are unlikely so seed cycling is unnecessary. For women whose hormone levels are imbalanced, seed cycling is unlikely to be the best way to improve this imbalance, and can actually over-complicate things.

There are no clinical studies showing any benefits of seed cycling on hormone balance and, while selenium, zinc and vitamin E are certainly important nutrients for fertility, there is no evidence that getting these nutrients from seeds over other foods is beneficial.

What are my recommendations?

I do not recommend seed cycling, simply because there is no evidence that even remotely suggests it is beneficial. I have also had patients come to me who have been advised to practise seed cycling and as a result have seen their stress and anxiety levels rise due to forgetting to have seeds on certain days, having to go through the process of grinding their seeds, and trying to remember what seeds they should be having at what point of their cycle. We know that stress is counterproductive to fertility and, if the intervention is not evidence-based, the level of stress it brings to some people is even more counterproductive.

That is not to say that including seeds in your diet is a waste of time, though; it isn't. Seeds are an excellent source of many nutrients important for fertility, and as I've mentioned in the micronutrient section of Chapter 13 (see page 158), I always recommend my male patients include seeds on a regular basis due to their high zinc content. They are also rich in that all important fibre, and contain many other micronutrients and components that are important, not just for fertility but for general health. So, including them regularly in your diet is a really positive thing, but it doesn't need to be regimented. Just adding them into your breakfast, or your smoothie/plant-based yoghurt, or any way you enjoy eating them, is perfectly fine. You don't need to worry if you don't manage to include them every day, just think about having them as part of a balanced plant-based diet.

Eating a pineapple after embryo transfer will aid implantation

This appears to be a popular thought among the IVF community and you can find countless social media posts extolling the virtues of pineapple (especially the core) consumption in the days pre and post embryo transfer. The thought is that, as bromelain, the enzyme in pineapple which is concentrated mainly in the core, has been shown to act as a mild blood thinner, this may aid implantation.

So, what does the science say?

There is no evidence that bromelain can be used as an effective measure in aiding implantation. However, a review of research into this showed that it might have mild blood-thinning actions,[1] and a more recent review found that it is likely to exert anti-inflammatory properties, including reducing the damaging effects of AGEs on cells.[2] This second review also agreed with the previous review that it might have blood thinning actions.

So, what do I recommend?

As the flesh of a pineapple actually contains very little bromelain, even if the evidence pointed to benefits of eating the enzyme for implantation, which it doesn't, it would likely have little effect. Bromelain is concentrated in the core and, although some of you may enjoy eating something that tough and fibrous, others (including myself) may not.

However, pineapple is a fruit, and we know that a variety of fruit and vegetables are beneficial to fertility. In addition, there are benefits to reducing the damaging effects of AGEs, so if you would like to add pineapple into your diet, it is a personal decision. Just be mindful though that, despite the many exaggerated claims on social media, it has not been shown to improve pregnancy outcomes.

Protein needs are higher during fertility treatment and protein powders are unnecessary

There are no guidelines to say that protein needs increase during fertility treatment. However, it is still really important to meet your daily needs.

Even if you are needing to eat much higher intakes of protein, as we have seen it is still possible to do this on a plant-based diet without the need for protein powders. The food-first approach is always preferable and, as long as a varied diet is being followed, taking protein powders is unnecessary. As I explained in Chapter 13, protein is everywhere and you only need to look at the protein table (Table 4, page 132) again to see just how much whole plant foods contain. This aside, there are a few reasons I do not generally advise my patients take protein powder, with one being the potential risk of contamination.

In 2020, the Clean Label Project released a report on the levels of toxins in protein powders after looking at 134 products and screening them for 130 types of toxin.[3] The report found that the majority of plant-based protein powders were contaminated with heavy metals, bisphenol-A, also known as BPA, pesticides or other contaminants associated with an increased risk of certain chronic diseases. However, the report has to be taken with a pinch of salt as the study was not submitted for peer review, which is a really important step in the development process of any scientific paper. The report states that the contaminants were 'detectable' in the protein powders; however, this does not necessarily mean they were found in levels harmful to human health. It's important to remember that heavy metals occur in the earth's crust and its soil so it is unsurprising that plant-based protein powders were found to have the highest levels of 'contamination.' The fact that over 50% of the powders tested were found to contain traces of BPA is more concerning as this means BPA is likely a component of the packaging and is leaching into the powder.

If you have PCOS or endometriosis, or are looking to optimise your fertility, it is a good idea to reduce your risk of exposure to BPA and look to minimise exposure to pesticides, so getting protein from whole food sources and thoroughly washing fruit and vegetables will help you to do this. You do not need to buy organic fruit and vegetables unless you prefer to and can afford it, as washing your produce well will remove any pesticide residues on the surface.

Aside from the potential contamination risk of BPA, protein powders are a processed food and some contain a long list of ingredients, including sunflower oil, gums, sweeteners and anti-caking agents. Also, unless you are exercising above a moderate rate for several hours a week, your protein needs will not be significantly increased and you will not need the addition of protein powders. It is much better in terms of nutrient content, avoiding unnecessary additives, and also for gut health to choose whole foods over protein powders, and also much better for your pocket too.

20

What supplements should I be taking?

Too often I see women or couples coming to clinic who have been advised by unqualified individuals to take a long list of supplements, some of which are herbal. The problem with taking herbal medications is that it is sometimes not clear what is actually in them and sometimes they may do more harm than good.

I do not routinely recommend a prenatal supplement marketed for this purpose as it very much depends on the quality of your diet. If you are eating plenty of fruit and vegetables, good quality carbohydrates and a high proportion overall of plant foods, you are unlikely to need the vast majority of nutrients contained in a multivitamin.

Also beware of supplements that promise to result in pregnancy. There are a lot of these out there and I have read the contents on their websites. Frankly, it is shocking. They look legit and they quote the science, but when you look into it either the research is massively flawed or they have simply made it up! They also make their products look even more appealing by having 'patient success stories', which of course anyone struggling to conceive will be drawn to. I am certain that the majority of these patients do not exist and, if they do, there are likely to be many more reasons behind their success than simply the supplement. Bottom line? If it looks too good to be true, avoid.

So, what do I recommend?

Again, what I recommend very much depends on overall diet quality, but there are some supplements that are really important for everyone trying to conceive, and I will split them into male, female and unisex categories.

Female

Folic acid

Folate or folic acid is non-negotiable as it really is so important for the health of your baby. Everyone trying to conceive should take a daily supplement. For those of you taking VEG1, which is a popular vegan supplement, you will need to take an additional folic acid supplement to make up the deficit as VEG1 only contains 200 mcg. As folic acid supplements come in 400 mcg doses, this means you will be taking 600 mcg in total, but this is absolutely fine, and actually many studies looking at the benefits of folic acid supplementation use slightly higher doses than the standard 400 mcg. For women with any of the underlying health problems I have mentioned in the folate section (see page 137), please do speak with your GP to see if you need the much higher dose of 5 mg daily.

Co-enzyme Q10 (CoQ10)

CoQ10 is not something I recommend routinely, but there is evidence that it may improve egg and embryo quality in women trying to conceive later in life. Our bodies produce CoQ10 naturally, but as we age our production naturally reduces. This is significant as CoQ 10 has antioxidant properties and is involved in protecting a woman's eggs from oxidative stress.[1] A recent review of five clinical trials found that supplementing women undergoing fertility treatment with CoQ10 resulted in an increase in clinical pregnancies when compared with those who were not supplemented. This applied to women with PCOS and poor ovarian response also.[2]

Increasing dietary sources is important and it is possible to meet your needs via food alone, but if a patient who is in their 30s or 40s would like to take a supplement, I support this. Dietary sources include soya foods, legumes, broccoli, strawberries, oranges, nuts (especially peanuts, pistachio and walnuts) and sesame seeds.

Dehydroepiandrosterone (or the much simpler abbreviation, DHEA)

DHEA is a steroid hormone produced naturally in the body that can be used to make other hormones, including testosterone and oestrogen. As it is involved in ovarian follicle development and oocyte quality, and because levels diminish with age, research has looked into whether it may be a beneficial supplement for women with poor ovarian reserves.

A recent systematic review and meta-analysis found that supplementing women with DHEA who had poor ovarian reserves during fertility treatment was associated with better outcomes and recommended this should be part of treatment protocol.[3] Many of my patients who have been through, or who are going through, IVF have been recommended this supplement by their team, but I would always advise anyone thinking about trying it to speak with their doctor first as it should not just be taken routinely.

Male

Co-enzyme Q10 (CoQ10)

Again, CoQ10 is not something I routinely recommend for men but there is evidence that it may help maintain the energy system of sperm and improve sperm quality, including improvements in motility and sperm concentration.[5] Supplementation has been shown to increase CoQ10 in the sperm, but the optimum dose has yet to be confirmed as different studies used different doses. The majority of studies have used 200 mg; however, benefits were seen at much lower doses, of 20-40 mg, and some studies have used much higher quantities. Supplements are available to buy at various doses but, based on the evidence, 100-200 mg daily appears to be optimal for those who are interested in trying CoQ10, but no higher than 600 mg. As for women, I would also highlight the importance of including regular food sources (soya foods, legumes, broccoli, strawberries, oranges, nuts and sesame seeds) and ideally increasing intakes of these first before resorting to a supplement.

Carnitine

I am including carnitine here because I have been asked many times whether an L-carnitine supplement should be taken to improve male fertility. Carnitine is derived from amino acids (remember, these are the building blocks of protein), and studies have shown it may play an important part in male fertility, but more research is needed. You can buy supplements which some of you may be familiar with, but you won't be surprised to hear that I don't routinely recommend men take these as I always advocate the food-first approach.

We don't actually need to consume carnitine via food or supplements because our liver and kidneys make enough from the amino acids lysine and methionine, both of which you can find in good amounts in plant foods. Legumes are great sources of lysine, and methionine is abundant in grain and vegetables, so, as is always the case, as long as you are eating a varied whole food plant-based diet, you will consume enough of these amino acids. There are some exceptions to this, which include those with chronic kidney or liver disease, or those taking certain medications. This includes long-term use of some antibiotics that may interfere with carnitine absorption, but for the vast majority of us there is no cause for concern. Even for those who may be deficient in carnitine, there have been no reported cases of illness associated with this.

Studies suggest that carnitine may be an important compound for treating male infertility as the concentration of it in the seminal fluid has been shown to be directly related to sperm count and motility. One study suggested that supplementation of 3 g per day for four months might improve sperm quality, with specific effects on concentration and motility.[4] However, a more recent clinical trial showed no improvements in sperm quality when infertile men were given 3 g per day for just under six months.[5] This demonstrates that more research is needed before any recommendations can be made. It is also important to know that supplements of around 3 g per day are associated with gastrointestinal symptoms like nausea, cramps, diarrhoea and also a fishy body odour. I would advise you to ensure you are eating plenty of legumes, grain and vegetables rather than taking a daily pill, at least until we have more evidence showing that it can help.

Unisex

Vitamin D

As I've already discussed in the micronutrient chapter, vitamin D supplementation is mandatory during the winter months to prevent deficiency, and all year around for certain groups (see page 152). During the summer months, I recommend a supplement to anyone who is not getting adequate sunlight daily, and this could apply to you if you are working in an office or from home and are not managing to get outside during the day. I always recommend a brisk 15-20 minute walk on your lunch break if possible, not only to get your vitamin D but to have a break from your work environment and to move your body, but I appreciate this is not always possible.

Basically, if you feel you are not getting enough sunshine during the summer months it is sensible to take a 20-50 mcg daily supplement.

Vitamin B12

Everyone on a plant-based diet should be taking a B12 supplement. It really is non-negotiable. I know there are fortified foods and if you are a lover of nutritional yeast and drink enough fortified milk it is possible in theory to meet your needs. However, it is difficult to make sure you are consistently consuming enough every day, especially when you go away for the weekend or go on holiday for longer. I have also spoken to GP colleagues who report that, despite meeting requirements with fortified food sources, many of their patients who were not also supplementing have been found to have B12 deficiency. Usually they have presented with extreme fatigue and, in some, tingling sensations in their fingers. It is for this reason that I advise everyone on a plant-based diet to supplement, regardless of their dietary intake.

Omega-3 fatty acids

We know that omega-3s are important for sperm health, and for women they may be more important for those trying to conceive later in life – that is, from around age 37 and above. However, as omega 3s play such key roles in the body, it may be beneficial for men and women to take a 400-500 mg supplement daily, in addition to including regular chia/ground flax and hemp, walnuts and other sources, as previously detailed.

Iodine

All men and women trying to conceive, and actually all plant-based eaters, should be taking a daily iodine supplement, with the iodine coming from potassium iodide or potassium iodate (you will see this stated in the ingredients). A tolerable upper limit has been set at 600 mcg by the European Food Safety Authority (EFSA) for all adults, including pregnant and breastfeeding women, but supplements should not exceed 150 mcg.

Other supplements

Of course, some may need additional supplements to those listed here depending on medical need or diet quality, but generally supplementation really is minimal for those trying to conceive. You should not be spending a fortune and taking supplements far in excess of what I have discussed here. If you are, please do speak to your doctor or dietitian for advice.

Final word

I really hope that you have enjoyed reading this book and now feel more confident in knowing how to work towards optimising both your and, if applicable, your partner's reproductive health. Never let a diagnosis of infertility make you give up because there is so much that can be done in terms of lifestyle changes to improve egg and sperm quality and get your body into fight mode to beat that diagnosis. Of course, not everyone who struggles to conceive will win the battle and that breaks my heart because everyone who wants to be a parent should get that opportunity.

For those of you who have suffered a pregnancy loss, please hear me when I say it is not your fault. So many women blame themselves for miscarrying, but nothing could be further from the truth and blaming yourself at a time when you need kindness and understanding will only make the process harder. Around 15% of clinically recognised pregnancies end in miscarriage, which is about one in six, and about 3% of these are recurrent miscarriage, which is defined as experiencing two or more miscarriages. In other words, miscarriage is really common so the fact that it is rarely spoken about is in stark contrast. I was greatly saddened to find out a few years ago how many people I knew had suffered one or more miscarriages. It still seems to be a taboo subject, but this needs to change because not only does it make people believe that miscarriage actually isn't that common, but it can prevent those who have experienced a pregnancy loss talking openly about it.

A woman may miscarry at four weeks or 16 weeks, but the impact is the same and should never be trivialised. Unfortunately, there are many misconceptions about miscarriage and these can cause so much damage, leaving women and their partners reluctant to seek help and support. Miscarriage is not caused by lifting something heavy, or having a few alcoholic drinks before you realised you were pregnant, or having previously had a sexually transmitted disease, or abortion. Believing these myths and not seeking the help you need can lead to grief not being fully addressed; this in turn can have psychological consequences. This can affect not only your mental health but also your physical health and your relationship, so it is vital to have a solid support network around you and also to seek professional help if you need it.

My sole aim in writing this book has always been to help as many couples and individuals as I can to be successful in their dreams of becoming parents. Not one piece of information in this book is cherry picked or, worse, made up. It is all evidence-based and I have spent hundreds of hours researching every part of this book to give you the most up-to-date information out there in the science space. I mentioned right at the beginning that I don't want to give anyone false hope. I know there is no guarantee that making positive dietary and lifestyle changes will result in a clinical pregnancy and birth, but I strongly believe that a little bit of hope is a positive thing. So many of my patients have come to see me feeling despondent and that they have lost that fight after struggling to conceive for such a long time. Some have gone through multiple miscarriages, others rounds of IVF treatment, and the one thing I always focus on is restoring that positive mindset; it really does make such a difference to how you feel physically as well as mentally.

Sending you all my love, positivity and strength, you've got this: ♥

Lisa x

References

Chapter 1: Infertility explained

1. Statistics O for N. Childbearing for women born in different years, England and Wales 2020 [Internet]. 2022 [cited 2022 Jul 30]. Available from: www.ons.gov.uk/peoplepopulationandcommunity/ birthsdeathsandmarriages/conceptionandfertilityrates/bulletins/ childbearingforwomenbornindifferentyearsenglandandwales/2020
2. Human Fertilisation and Embryology Authority. Fertility treatment 2019: trends and figures [Internet]. 2021 [cited 2022 Aug 1]. Available from: www.hfea.gov.uk/about-us/publications/research-and-data/ fertility-treatment-2019-trends-and-figures/
3. Human Fertilisation and Embryology Authority. IVF treatment safer, more available and more successful than ever before, new report shows [Internet]. 2018. [cited 2022 Aug 1]. Available from: www.hfea.gov.uk/ about-us/news-and-press-releases/2018-news-and-press-releases/ press-release-ivf-treatment-safer-more-available-and-more- successful-than-ever-before-new-report-shows/

Chapter 2: The male reproductive system

1. Culley L, Hudson N, Lohan M. Where are all the men? the marginalization of men in social scientific research on infertility. In: Reproductive BioMedicine Online. 2013; 27(3): 225-235 DOI: 10.1016/j.rbmo.2013.06.009
2. Leaver RB. Male infertility: An overview of causes and treatment options. *British Journal of Nursing* 2016; 25: S35-S40. DOI: 10.12968/bjon.2016.25.18.S35
3. Hanna E, Gough B. Experiencing male infertility: A review of the qualitative research literature. *SAGE Open* 2015; 5(4): 1-9. DOI: 10.1177/2158244015610319
4. Tiegs AW, Landis J, Garrido N, Scott RT, Hotaling JM. Total Motile Sperm Count Trend Over Time: Evaluation of Semen Analyses From 119,972 Men From Subfertile Couples. *Urology* 2019; 132: 109-116. DOI: 10.1016/j.urology.2019.06.038

5. Mann U, Shiff B, Patel P. Reasons for worldwide decline in male fertility. *Current Opinion in Urology* 2020; 30: 296-301. DOI: 10.1097/MOU.0000000000000745

6. Agarwal A, Deepinder F, Sharma RK, Ranga G, Li J. Effect of cell phone usage on semen analysis in men attending infertility clinic: an observational study. *Fertil Steril* 2007; 89: 124–128. doi: 10.1016/j.fertnstert.2007.01.166Kesari KK and Agarwal A, Henkel R. Radiations and male fertility. *Reprod Biol Endocrinol* 2018; 16: 118. DOI: 10.1186/s12958-018-0431-1

7. Ostfeld RJ, Allen KE, Aspry K, Brandt EJ, Spitz A, Liberman J, et al. Vasculogenic Erectile Dysfunction: The Impact of Diet and Lifestyle. *American Journal of Medicine* 2021; 134(3): 310-316. DOI: 10.1016/j.amjmed.2020.09.033

8. Li N, Wu X, Zhuang W, Xia L, Chen Y, Zhao R, et al. Soy and Isoflavone Consumption and Multiple Health Outcomes: Umbrella Review of Systematic Reviews and Meta-Analyses of Observational Studies and Randomized Trials in Humans. *Molecular Nutrition and Food Research* 2020; 64(4): e1900751. DOI: 10.1002/mnfr.201900751

9. Kresch E, Blachman-Braun R, Nackeeran S, Kuchakulla M, Ramasamy R. PD20-05 plant based diets are associated with decreased risk of erectile dysfunction. *J Urol* 2021; 206(Supplement 3): e368-e369. DOI: 10.1097/ju.0000000000002009.05

Chapter 4: PCOS (polycystic ovary syndrome)

1. Teede HJ, Misso ML, Costello MF, Dokras A, Laven J, Moran L, et al. Recommendations from the international evidence-based guideline for the assessment and management of polycystic ovary syndrome. *Hum Reprod* 2018; 33(9): 1602-1618. DOI: 10.1093/humrep/dey256

2. Jiskoot G, Benneheij SH, Beerthuizen A, De Niet JE, De Klerk C, Timman R, et al. A three-component cognitive behavioural lifestyle program for preconceptional weight-loss in women with polycystic ovary syndrome (PCOS): A protocol for a randomized controlled trial. Reprod Health 2017; 14(1): 34. DOI: 10.1186/s12978-017-0295-4

3. Tanvir K, Rahman ML. Pregnancy Complications in Women with PCOS: A Meta-Analysis. *Dhaka Univ J Sci* 2021; 69(2): 82-87. DOI: 10.3329/dujs.v69i2.56487

4. Ye W, Xie T, Song Y, Zhou L. The role of androgen and its related signals in PCOS. *Journal of Cellular and Molecular Medicine* 2021; 25: 1825-1837. DOI: 10.1111/jcmm.16205

5. Stepto NK, Hiam D, Gibson-Helm M, Cassar S, Harrison CL, Hutchison SK, et al. Exercise and insulin resistance in PCOS: Muscle insulin signalling and fibrosis. *Endocr Connect* 2020; 9(4): 346-359. DOI: 10.1530/EC-19-0551

6. Kokanall D, Karaca M, Ozak it G, Elmas B, Üstün YE. Serum Vitamin D Levels in Fertile and Infertile Women with Polycystic Ovary Syndrome. *Geburtshilfe Frauenheilkd* 2019; 79(5): 510-516. DOI: 10.1055/a-0828-7798

7. Bosdou JK, Konstantinidou E, Anagnostis P, Kolibianakis EM, Goulis DG. Vitamin D and obesity: Two interacting players in the field of infertility. *Nutrients* 2019; 11: 1455. DOI: 10.3390/nu11071455

8. Jiskoot G, Dietz de Loos A, Beerthuizen A, Timman R, Busschbach J, Laven J. Long-term effects of a three-component lifestyle intervention on emotional well-being in women with Polycystic Ovary Syndrome (PCOS): A secondary analysis of a randomized controlled trial. *PLoS One* 2020; 15(6): e0233876. DOI: 10.1371/journal.pone.0233876

9. Louwers Y V., Rayner NW, Herrera BM, Stolk L, Groves CJ, Barber TM, et al. BMI-associated alleles do not constitute risk alleles for polycystic ovary syndrome independently of BMI: A case-control study. *PLoS One* 2014; 9(1): e87335. DOI: 10.1371/journal.pone.0087335

10. Cutler DA, Pride SM, Cheung AP. Low intakes of dietary fiber and magnesium are associated with insulin resistance and hyperandrogenism in polycystic ovary syndrome: A cohort study. *Food Sci Nutr* 2019; 7(4): 1426-1437. DOI: 10.1002/fsn3.977

11. Gallager W. Apple Women's Health Study uncovers impact of PCOS on other medical issues *AppleInsider* 28 February 2022. https://appleinsider.com/articles/22/02/28/apple-womens-health-study-uncovers-impact-of-pcos-on-other-medical-issues Accessed 24th November 2022

12. Kamenov Z, Gateva A. Inositols in pcos. *Molecules* 2020; 25: 5566. DOI: 10.3390/molecules25235566

13. Roseff S, Montenegro M. Inositol treatment for PCOS should be science-based and not arbitrary. *International Journal of Endocrinology* 2020; 2020: 5566. DOI: 10.1155/2020/6461254

14. Unfer V, Facchinetti F, Orrù B, Giordani B, Nestler J. Myo-inositol effects in women with PCOS: A meta-analysis of randomized controlled trials. *Endocr Connect* 2017; 6(8):647-658. DOI: 10.1530/EC-17-0243

Chapter 5: Endometriosis

1. Bonocher CM, Montenegro ML, Rosa e Silva JC, Ferriani RA, Meola J. Endometriosis and physical exercises: A systematic review. *Reproductive Biology and Endocrinology* 2014; 12: 4. DOI: 10.1186/1477-7827-12-4

2. Scutiero G, Iannone P, Bernardi G, Bonaccorsi G, Spadaro S, Volta CA, et al. Oxidative Stress and Endometriosis: A Systematic Review of the Literature. *Oxidative Medicine and Cellular Longevity* 2017; 2017. DOI: 10.1155/2017/7265238

3. Jurkiewicz-Przondziono J, Lemm M, Kwiatkowska-Pamula A, Ziółłko E, Wójtowicz MK. Influence of diet on the risk of developing endometriosis. *Ginekol Pol* 2017; 88(2): 96-102. DOI: 10.5603/GP.a2017.0017

4. Qi X, Zhang W, Ge M, Sun Q, Peng L, Cheng W, et al. Relationship Between Dairy Products Intake and Risk of Endometriosis: A Systematic Review and Dose-Response Meta-Analysis. *Frontiers in Nutrition* 2021; 8: 701860. DOI: 10.3389/fnut.2021.701860

5. Harris HR, Chavarro JE, Malspeis S, Willett WC, Missmer SA. Dairy-food, calcium, magnesium, and vitamin D intake and endometriosis: A prospective cohort study. *Am J Epidemiol* 2013; 177(5): 420-430. DOI: 10.1093/aje/kws247

6. Harris HR, Eke AC, Chavarro JE, Missmer SA. Fruit and vegetable consumption and risk of endometriosis. *Hum Reprod* 2018; 33(4): 715-727. DOI: 10.1093/humrep/dey014

7. Chavarro JE, Rich-Edwards JW, Rosner BA, Willett WC. Protein intake and ovulatory infertility. *Am J Obstet Gynecol* 2008; 198(2): 210. e1-210.e.7. DOI: 10.1016/j.ajog.2007.06.057

8. Zhao G, Shi Y, Gong C, Liu T, Nan W, Ma L, et al. Curcumin Exerts Antinociceptive Effects in Cancer-Induced Bone Pain via an Endogenous Opioid Mechanism. *Front Neurosci* 2021; 15: 696861. DOI: 10.3389/fnins.2021.696861

9. Jamali N, Adib-Hajbaghery M, Soleimani A. The effect of curcumin ointment on knee pain in older adults with osteoarthritis: A randomized placebo trial. *BMC Complement Med Ther* 2020; 20(1): 305. DOI: 10.1186/s12906-020-03105-0

10. Tennfjord MK, Gabrielsen R, Tellum T. Effect of physical activity and exercise on endometriosis-associated symptoms: a systematic review. *BMC Womens Health* 2021; 21(1): 355. DOI: 10.1186/s12905-021-01500-4

Chapter 6: Inequalities in fertility care

1. Bärnreuther S. Racializing infertility: How South/Asian-ness has been constituted as an independent risk factor in infertility research and IVF practice. *Soc Sci Med* 2021; 280: DOI: 10.1016/j.socscimed.2021.114008.
2. Mahmud G, Lopez Bernal A, Yudkin P, Ledger W, Barlow DH. A controlled assessment of the in vitro fertilization performance of British women of indian origin compared with white women. *Fertil Steril* 1995; 64(1): 103-106. DOI: 10.1016/s0015-0282(16)57663-8
3. Galic I, Negris O, Warren C, et al. Disparitites in access to fertility care: who's in and who's out. *Epidemiology* 2020; 2(1): 109–17. Available from: https://pubmed.ncbi.nlm.nih.gov/34223281/#:~:text=Disparities in access to fertility care%3A who%27s in,socioeconomic disparities exist among fertility patients accessing care.
4. Nuriddin A, Mooney GWA. Reckoning with histories of medical racism and violence in the USA. *Lancet* 2020; 396(10256): 949–951. Available from: https://reader.elsevier.com/reader/sd/pii/S0140673620320328?token=17A606875463DF44BA45FAFF4273B4F1CBCACFB3B39C079ADACDA49070E7D633819699FB94198B4BF7CB95CB842607C8&originRegion=eu-west-1&originCreation=20220728150656
5. NHS. Race and health observatory. www.nhsrho.org (accessed 18 January 2023)
6. Human Fertilisation and Embryology Authority. Ethnic diversity in fertility treatment 2018 [Internet]. 2018 [cited 2022 Aug 1]. Available from: www.hfea.gov.uk/about-us/publications/research-and-data/ethnic-diversity-in-fertility-treatment-2018/
7. Gameiro S, El Refaie E, De Guevara BB, Payson A. Women from diverse minority ethnic or religious backgrounds desire more infertility education and more culturally and personally sensitive fertility care. *Hum Reprod* 2019; 34(9): 1735-1745. DOI: 10.1093/humrep/dez156
8. Tonkin. T. Racism an issue in the NHS, finds survey [Internet]. BMA 2022 [cited 2022 Jul 29]. Available from: www.bma.org.uk/news-and-opinion/racism-an-issue-in-nhs-finds-survey
9. Jackson-Bey T, Morris J, Jasper E, et al. Systematic review of racial and ethnic disparities in reproductive endocrinology and infertility: where do we stand today? *Fertil Steril* 2021; 2(3): 169–188. Available from: https://www.fertstertreviews.org/article/S2666-5719(21)00011-6/fulltext
10. Quenby S, Gallos I, Dhillon-Smith RDD-SR, et al. Miscarriage matters: the epidemiological, physical, psychological and economic costs of early pregnancy loss. *Lancet* 2021; 397(10285): 1658–1667.

11. Maxwell E, Mathews M, Mulay S. More than a biological condition: The heteronormative framing of infertility. *Canadian Journal of Bioethics* 2018; 1: 63-66. DOI: 10.7202/1058269AR.

Chapter 7: The preconception period

1. Billah MM, Khatiwada S, Morris MJ, Maloney CA. Effects of paternal overnutrition and interventions on future generations. *International Journal of Obesity* 2022; 46: 901-917. DOI: 10.1038/s41366-021-01042-7

2. Shawe J, Ceulemans D, Akhter Z, Neff K, Hart K, Heslehurst N, et al. Pregnancy after bariatric surgery: Consensus recommendations for periconception, antenatal and postnatal care. *Obesity Reviews* 2019; 20: 1507-1522. DOI: 10.1111/obr.12927.

3. WHO. Obesity and overweight. 9 June 2021 www.who.int/news-room/fact-sheets/detail/obesity-and-overweight

4. Stephenson J, Heslehurst N, Hall J, Schoenaker DAJM, Hutchinson J, Cade JE, et al. Before the beginning: nutrition and lifestyle in the preconception period and its importance for future health. *Lancet* 2018; 391: DOI: 10.1016/s0140-6736(18)30311-8

5. Van der Steeg JW, Steures P, Eijkemans M, et al. Obesity affects spontaneous pregnancy chances in subfertile, ovulatory women. *Hum Rep* 2008; 23(2): 324-328. DOI:10.1093/humrep/dem371

6. Sermondade N, Faure C, Fezeu L, Shayeb AG, Bonde JP, Jensen TK, et al. BMI in relation to sperm count: An updated systematic review and collaborative meta-analysis. *Hum Reprod Update* 2013; 19(3): 221-231. DOI: 10.1093/humupd/dms050

7. Zhang Y, Zhang J, Zhao J, Hong X, Zhang H, Dai Q, et al. Couples' prepregnancy body mass index and time to pregnancy among those attempting to conceive their first pregnancy. *Fertil Steril* 2020; 114(5): 1067-1075. DOI: 10.1016/j.fertnstert.2020.05.041

8. Sallmén M, Sandler DP, Hoppin JA, Blair A, Baird DD. Reduced fertility among overweight and obese men. *Epidemiology* 2006; 17(5): 520-523. DOI: 10.1097/01.ede.0000229953.76862.e5

9. Han Z, Mulla S B. Maternal underweight and the risk of pre-term birth and low birth rate: a systematic review and meta-analyses. *Int J Epidemiol* 2011; 40(1): 65–101.

10. Håkonsen L, Thulstrup A, Aggerholm A, Olsen J, Bonde J, Andersen C, et al. Does weight loss improve semen quality and reproductive hormones? results from a cohort of severely obese men. *Reprod Health* 2011; 8(1): 24. DOI: 10.1186/1742-4755-8-24

Chapter 8: Oxidative stress

1. Agarwal A, Gupta S, Sharma RK. Role of oxidative stress in female reproduction. *Reproductive Biology and Endocrinology* 2005; 3: Article 28. DOI: 10.1186/1477-7827-3-28

2. Adewoyin M, Ibrahim M, Roszaman R, Isa M, Alewi N, Rafa A, et al. Male Infertility: The Effect of Natural Antioxidants and Phytocompounds on Seminal Oxidative Stress. *Diseases* 2017; 5(1): 9. DOI: 10.3390/diseases5010009.

3. Lateef OM, Akintubosun MO. Sleep and reproductive health. *Journal of Circadian Rhythms* 2020; 18: 1-11. DOI: 10.5334/jcr.190.

4. Aoun A, El Khoury V, Malakieh R. Can nutrition help in the treatment of infertility? *Preventive Nutrition and Food Science* 2021; 26(2): 109-120. DOI: 10.3746/pnf.2021.26.2.109

Chapter 9: Animal foods and effects on fertility

1. Chavarro JE, Rich-Edwards JW, Rosner BA, Willett WC. Protein intake and ovulatory infertility. *Am J Obstet Gynecol* 2008; 198(2): P210. E1-210.E7. DOI: 10.1016/j.ajog.2007.06.057

2. Braga DPAF, Halpern G, Setti AS, Figueira RCS, Iaconelli A, Borges E. The impact of food intake and social habits on embryo quality and the likelihood of blastocyst formation. *Reprod Biomed Online* 2015; 31(1): 30-38. DOI: 10.1016/j.rbmo.2015.03.007

3. Van TTH, Yidana Z, Smooker PM, Coloe PJ. Antibiotic use in food animals worldwide, with a focus on Africa: Pluses and minuses. *Journal of Global Antimicrobial Resistance* 2020; 20: 170-177. DOI: 10.1016/j.jgar.2019.07.031

4. Mallidis C, Agbaje IM, Rogers DA, Glenn J V., Pringle R, Atkinson AB, et al. Advanced glycation end products accumulate in the reproductive tract of men with diabetes. *Int J Androl* 2009; 32(4): 295-305. DOI: 10.1111/j.1365-2605.2007.00849.x

5. Setti AS, Halpern G, Braga DP de AF, Iaconelli A, Borges E. Maternal lifestyle and nutritional habits are associated with oocyte quality and ICSI clinical outcomes. *Reprod Biomed Online* 2021; 44(2): 370-379. DOI: 10.1016/j.rbmo.2021.08.025

6. Chavarro JE, Rich-Edwards JW, Rosner BA, Willett WC. Dietary fatty acid intakes and the risk of ovulatory infertility. *Am J Clin Nutr* 2007; 85(1): 231-237. DOI: 10.1093/ajcn/85.1.231

7. Smith M, Love DC, Rochman CM, Neff RA. Microplastics in Seafood

and the Implications for Human Health. *Current Environmental Health Reports* 2018; 5: 375-386. DOI: 10.1007/s40572-018-0206-z

Chapter 11: Phytonutrients

1. Pérez-Jiménez J, Neveu V, Vos F, Scalbert A. Identification of the 100 richest dietary sources of polyphenols: An application of the Phenol-Explorer database. *Eur J Clin Nutr* 2010; 64: S112-S120. DOI: 10.1038/ejcn.2010.221

Chapter 12: The gut microbiota

1. Silva YP, Bernardi A, Frozza RL. The Role of Short-Chain Fatty Acids From Gut Microbiota in Gut-Brain Communication. *Frontiers in Endocrinology* 2020; 11: Article 25. DOI: 10.3389/fendo.2020.00025
2. WHO. Cancer: Carcinogenicity of the consumption of red and processed meat. WHO 26 October 2015. www.who.int/news-room/questions-and-anwers/item/cancer-carcinogeicity-of-the-consumption-of-red-meat-and-prcessed-meat
3. Lee KA, Luong MK, Shaw H, Nathan P, Bataille V, Spector TD. The gut microbiome: what the oncologist ought to know. *British Journal of Cancer* 2021; 125: 1197-1209. DOI: 10.1038/s41416-021-01467-x
4. Rezac S, Kok CR, Heermann M, Hutkins R. Fermented foods as a dietary source of live organisms. *Frontiers in Microbiology* 2018; 9: Article 1785. DOI: 10.3389/fmicb.2018.01785
5. Li N, Wu X, Zhuang W, Xia L, Chen Y, Zhao R, et al. Soy and Isoflavone Consumption and Multiple Health Outcomes: Umbrella Review of Systematic Reviews and Meta-Analyses of Observational Studies and Randomized Trials in Humans. *Molecular Nutrition and Food Research* 2020; 64: e1900751. DOI: 10.1002/mnfr.201900751

Chapter 13: Pillar 1 – Nutrition

1. Setti AS, Halpern G, Braga DP de AF, Iaconelli A, Borges E. Maternal lifestyle and nutritional habits are associated with oocyte quality and ICSI clinical outcomes. *Reprod Biomed Online* 2021; 44 (2): 370-379. DOI: 10.1016/j.rbmo.2021.08.025
2. Kljajic M, Kasoha M, Seyfried S, Solomayer E-F. A Preliminary Study:

Impact of the vegan diet on sperm quality and sperm oxidative stress values. In: *Kongressabstracts zur Tagung 2020 der Deutschen Gesellschaft für Gynäkologie und Geburtshilfe (DGGG)*. 2020.14 (4): 365-371. DOI: 10.4103/jhrs.jhrs_90_21

3. Shevlyakov A, Nikogosov D, Stewart LA, Toribio-Mateas M. Reference values for intake of six types of soluble and insoluble fibre in healthy UK inhabitants based on the UK Biobank data. *Public Health Nutr* 2021; 25(5): 1-15. DOI: 10.1017/S1368980021002524

4. Pituch-Zdanowska A, Banaszkiewicz A, Albrecht P. The role of dietary fibre in inflammatory bowel disease. *Przeglad Gastroenterologiczny* 2015; 10 (3): 135-141. DOI: 10.5114/pg.2015.52753

5. Gaskins AJ, Chiu YH, Williams PL, Keller MG, Toth TL, Hauser R, et al. Maternal whole grain intake and outcomes of in vitro fertilization. *Fertil Steril* 2016; 105(6): 1503-1510.e4. DOI: 10.1016/j.fertnstert.2016.02.015

6. WHO. Nutrition: Trans fats [Internet] 2018 Available from: www.who. int/news-room/questions-and-answers/item/nutrition-trans-fat [cited 2022 Nov 4]

7. Chavarro J, Rich-Edwards J, Rosner B. Diet and Lifestyle in the Prevention of Ovulatory Disorder Infertility. *Obstetrics and Gynecology* 2007; 110(5): 1050-1058. DOI: 10.1097/01.AOG.0000287293.25465.e1

8. Chavarro JE, Rich-Edwards JW, Rosner BA, Willett WC. Protein intake and ovulatory infertility. *Am J Obstet Gynecol* 2008; 198(2): 210.e1-210. e7. DOI: 10.1016/j.ajog.2007.06.057

9. Innes JK, Calder PC. Omega-6 fatty acids and inflammation. *Prostaglandins Leukotrienes and Essential Fatty Acids* 2018; 132: 41-48. DOI: 10.1016/j.plefa.2018.03.004

10. Robbins WA, Xun L, FitzGerald LZ, Esguerra S, Henning SM, Carpenter CL. Walnuts improve semen quality in men consuming a western-style diet: Randomized control dietary intervention trial. *Biol Reprod* 2012; 87(4): 101, 1-8. DOI: 10.1095/biolreprod.112.101634

11. Falsig AML, Gleerup CS, Knudsen UB. The influence of omega-3 fatty acids on semen quality markers: a systematic PRISMA review. *Andrology* 2019; 7 (6): 794-803. DOI: 10.1111/andr.12649

12. Chiu YH, Karmon AE, Gaskins AJ, Arvizu M, Williams PL, Souter I, et al. Serum omega-3 fatty acids and treatment outcomes among women undergoing assisted reproduction. *Hum Reprod* 2018; 33(1): 156-165. DOI: 10.1093/humrep/dex335

13. Stanhiser J, Jukic AMZ, Steiner AZ. Serum omega-3 and omega-6 fatty acid concentrations and natural fertility. *Hum Reprod* 2021; 35(4): 950-957. DOI: 10.1093/humrep/dez305

14. Comerford KB, Ayoob KT, Murray RD, Atkinson SA. The role of avocados in maternal diets during the periconceptional period, pregnancy, and lactation. *Nutrients* 2016; 8: 313. DOI: 10.3390/nu8050313

15. Agostoni C, Galli C, Riva E, Risé P, Colombo C, Giovannini M, et al. Whole blood fatty acid composition at birth: From the maternal compartment to the infant. *Clin Nutr* 2011; 30(4): 503-505. DOI: 10.1016/j.clnu.2011.01.016

16. Agostoni C, Marangoni F, Stival G, Gatelli I, Pinto F, RisI P, et al. Whole blood fatty acid composition differs in term versus mildly preterm infants: Small versus matched appropriate for gestational age. *Pediatr Res* 2008; 64(3): 298-302. DOI: 10.1203/PDR.0b013331817d9c23

17. Gaskins AJ, Chavarro JE. Diet and fertility: a review. *American Journal of Obstetrics and Gynecology* 2018; 218(4). DOI: 10.1016/j.ajog.2017.08.010

18. Reed KE, Camargo J, Hamilton-Reeves J, Kurzer M, Messina M. Neither soy nor isoflavone intake affects male reproductive hormones: An expanded and updated meta-analysis of clinical studies. *Reproductive Toxicology* 2021; 100: 60-67. DOI: 10.1016/j.reprotox.2020.12.019

19. Chiu YH, Chavarro JE, Souter I. Diet and female fertility: doctor, what should I eat? *Fertility and Sterility* 2018; 110 (4): 560-569. DOI: 10.1016/j.fertnstert.2018.05.027

20. Rizzo G, Feraco A, Storz MA, Lombardo M. The role of soy and soy isoflavones on women's fertility and related outcomes: an update. *J Nutr Sci* 2022; 11: e17 1-17. doi.org/10.1017/jns.2022.15

21. House SH, Nichols JA, Rae S. Folates, folic acid and preconception care – a review. *JRSM Open* 2021; 12(5): 1-7. DOI: 10.1177/2054270420980875

22. Sullivan M, Murray T, Assefa H. Women with Methylenetetrahydrofolate Reductase Gene Polymorphism and the Need for Proper Periconceptional Folate Supplementation. *J Pharm Pharmacol* 2015; 3(5): 204-222. DOI: 10.17265/2328-2150/2015.05.002

23. Skoracka K, Ratajczak AE, Rychter AM, Dobrowolska A, Krela-Kaźmierczak I. Female Fertility and the Nutritional Approach: The Most Essential Aspects. *Advances in Nutrition* 2021; 12: 2372-2386. DOI: 10.1093/advances/nmab068

24. Balogun OO, da Silva Lopes K, Ota E, Takemoto Y, Rumbold A, Takegata M, et al. Vitamin supplementation for preventing miscarriage. *Cochrane Database of Systematic Reviews* 2016; 2016(5): CD004073. DOI: 10.1002/14651858.CD004073.pub4

25. Wong WY, Merkus HMWM, Thomas CMG, Menkveld R, Zielhuis GA,

Steegers-Theunissen RPM. Effects of folic acid and zinc sulfate on male factor subfertility: A double-blind, randomized, placebo-controlled trial. *Fertil Steril* 2002; 77(3): 491–498.

26. Salas-Huetos A, Rosique-Esteban N, Becerra-Tomás N, Vizmanos B, Bulló M, Salas-Salvadó J. The effect of nutrients and dietary supplements on sperm quality parameters: A systematic review andmeta-analysis of randomized clinical trials. *Advances in Nutrition* 2018; 9: 833-848. DOI: 10.1093/ADVANCES/NMY057

27. Schisterman EF, Sjaarda LA, Clemons T, Carrell DT, Perkins NJ, Johnstone E, et al. Effect of Folic Acid and Zinc Supplementation in Men on Semen Quality and Live Birth among Couples Undergoing Infertility Treatment: A Randomized Clinical Trial. *JAMA - J Am Med Assoc* 2020; 323(1): 35-48. DOI: 10.1001/jama.2019.18714

28. Isomah AC, Allison RO, Christian SG, Eze EM. Evaluation of Vitamin B_{12}, Folate, Haematological Parameters and Some Reproductive Hormones in Subjects Attending Fertility Centres in Port Harcourt. *Eur J Med Heal Sci* 2021; 3(4): 109-115. DOI: 10.24018/ejmed.2021.3.4.891

29. Vanderhout SM, Panah MR, Garcia-Bailo B, Grace-Farfaglia P, Samsel K, Dockray J, et al. Nutrition, genetic variation and male fertility. *Translational Andrology and Urology* 2021; 10(3): 1410-1431. DOI: 10.21037/tau-20-592

30. Adewoyin M, Ibrahim M, Roszaman R, Isa M, Alewi N, Rafa A, et al. Male Infertility: The Effect of Natural Antioxidants and Phytocompounds on Seminal Oxidative Stress. *Diseases* 2017; 5(1): 9. DOI: 10.3390/diseases5010009

31. Kazemi A, Ramezanzadeh F, Nasr-Esfahani MH. The relations between dietary antioxidant vitamins intake and oxidative stress in follicular fluid and ART outcomes. *Iran J Reprod Med* 2015; 13(9): 533-540.

32. Sharami SH, Bahadori MH, Fakor F, Mirblouk F, Kazemi S, Pourmarzi D, et al. Relationship between follicular fluid and serum levels of vitamin C and oocyte morphology and embryo quality in patients undergoing in vitro fertilization. *Int J Women's Heal Reprod Sci* 2017; 5(1): 41-46. DOI: 10.15296/ijwhr.2017.08

33. Bosdou JK, Konstantinidou E, Anagnostis P, Kolibianakis EM, Goulis DG. Vitamin D and obesity: Two interacting players in the field of infertility. *Nutrients* 2019; 11: 1455. DOI: 10.3390/nu11071455

34. Arab A, Hadi A, Moosavian SP, Askari G, Nasirian M. The association between serum vitamin D, fertility and semen quality: A systematic review and meta-analysis. *International Journal of Surgery* 2019; 71: 101-109. DOI: 10.1016/j.ijsu.2019.09.025

35. Bahadori MH, Sharami SH, Fakor F, Milani F, Pourmarzi D,

Dalil-Heirati SF. Level of Vitamin E in Follicular Fluid and Serum and Oocyte Morphology and Embryo Quality in Patients Undergoing IVF Treatment. *J Fam Reprod Heal* 2017; 11(2): 74-81.

36. Jouanne M, Oddoux S, Noël A, Voisin-Chiret AS. Nutrient requirements during pregnancy and lactation. *Nutrients* 2021; 13(2): 1-17. DOI: 10.3390/nu13020692

37. Qazi IH, Angel C, Yang H, Pan B, Zoidis E, Zeng CJ, et al. Selenium, selenoproteins, and female reproduction: A review. *Molecules* 2018; 23: 3053. DOI: 10.3390/molecules23123053

38. Duntas LH. Selenium and at-risk pregnancy: Challenges and controversies. *Thyroid Research* 2020; 13: 16. DOI: 10.1186/s13044-020-00090-x

39. Ahmadip S, Bashirip R, Ghadiri-Anarip A, Nadjarzadehp A. Antioxidant supplements and semen parameters: An evidence based review. *International Journal of Reproductive BioMedicine* 2016; 14:729-736. DOI: 10.29252/ijrm.14.12.729

40. Chatzicharalampous C, Jeelani R, Mikhael S, Aldhaheri S, Najeemudin S, Morris RT, et al. Zinc: an essential metal for maintenance of female fertility. *Fertil Steril* 2018; 109(3): e19. DOI: 10.1016/j.fertnstert.2018.02.043

41. Mills JL, Buck Louis GM, Kannan K, Weck J, Wan Y, Maisog J, et al. Delayed conception in women with low-urinary iodine concentrations: A population-based prospective cohort study. *Hum Reprod* 2018; 33(3): 426-433. DOI: 10.1093/humrep/dex379

42. Sun Y, Chen C, Liu GG, Wang M, Shi C, Yu G, et al. The association between iodine intake and semen quality among fertile men in China. *BMC Public Health* 2020; 20(1): 461. DOI: 10.1186/s12889-020-08547-2

43. Bouga M, Combet E. Emergence of seaweed and seaweed-containing foods in the uk: Focus on labeling, iodine content, toxicity and nutrition. *Foods* 2015; 4(2): 240-253. DOI: 10.3390/foods4020240

44. Tvrda E, Peer R, Sikka SC, Agarwal A. Iron and copper in male reproduction: a double-edged sword. *J Assist Reprod Genet* 2015; 32(1): 3-16. DOI: 10.1007/s10815-014-0344-7

45. Jiang X, Bar HY, Yan J, Jones S, Brannon PM, West AA, et al. A higher maternal choline intake among third-trimester pregnant women lowers placental and circulating concentrations of the antiangiogenic factor fms-like tyrosine kinase-1 (sFLT1). *FASEB J* 2013; 27(3): 1245-1253. DOI: 10.1096/fj.12-221648

46. National Institutes for Health. Choline Factsheet for Health Professionals [Internet]. 2022 [cited 2022 Jul 26]. Available from: https://ods.od.nih.gov/factsheets/Choline-HealthProfessional/

47. EFSA European Food Safety Authority [Internet]. 2019 [cited 2022 Jul 26]. p. 1–8. Available from: file:///C:/Users/tip-t/Downloads/DRVs_Adults.pdf

48. Melina BD and V. Becoming Vegan: the Complete Guide to Plant-Based Nutrition. US: Book Publishing Company; 2014.

49. Whitaker M. Calcium at fertilization and in early development. *Physiol Rev* 2006; 86(1): 25–88. DOI: 10.1152/physrev.00023.2005

50. López-Plaza B, Bermejo LM, Santurino C, Cavero-Redondo I, Álvarez-Bueno C, Gómez-Candela C. Milk and Dairy Product Consumption and Prostate Cancer Risk and Mortality: An Overview of Systematic Reviews and Meta-analyses. *Advances in Nutrition* 2019; 10: S212-S223. DOI: 10.1093/advances/nmz014

51. Vázquez-Fresno R, Rosana ARR, Sajed T, Onookome-Okome T, Wishart NA, Wishart DS. Herbs and Spices- Biomarkers of Intake Based on Human Intervention Studies - A Systematic Review. *Genes and Nutrition* 2019; 14: 18. DOI: 10.1186/s12263-019-0636-8

52. Pérez-Jiménez J, Neveu V, Vos F, Scalbert A. Identification of the 100 richest dietary sources of polyphenols: An application of the Phenol-Explorer database. *Eur J Clin Nutr* 2010; 64: S112-S120. DOI: 10.1038/ejcn.2010.221

Chapter 14: Pillar 2 – Exercise

1. Sharma R, Biedenharn KR, Fedor JM, Agarwal A. Lifestyle factors and reproductive health: Taking control of your fertility. *Reproductive Biology and Endocrinology* 2013; 11: 66. DOI: 10.1186/1477-7827-11-66

2. Agarwal A. Is There a Link between Exercise and Male Factor Infertility? *Open Reprod Sci J* 2011; 3(1): 105-113. DOI: 10.2174/1874255601103010105

3. Urso ML, Clarkson PM. Oxidative stress, exercise, and antioxidant supplementation. *Toxicology* 2003; 189: 41-54. DOI: 10.1016/S0300-483X(03)00151-3

4. Yavari A, Javadi M, Mirmiran P, Bahadoran Z. Exercise-induced oxidative stress and dietary antioxidants. *Asian Journal of Sports Medicine* 2015; 6: e24898. DOI: 10.5812/asjsm.24898

Chapter 15: Pillar 3 – Stress

1. Hill D, Conner M, Clancy F, Moss R, Wilding S, Bristow M, et al. Stress and eating behaviours in healthy adults: a systematic review and meta-analysis. *Health Psychol Rev* 2022; 16(2): 280-304.
   DOI: 10.1080/17437199.2021.1923406
2. Ilacqua A, Izzo G, Emerenziani G Pietro, Baldari C, Aversa A. Lifestyle and fertility: The influence of stress and quality of life on male fertility. *Reproductive Biology and Endocrinology* 2018; 16: 115.
   DOI: 10.1186/s12958-018-0436-9
3. Friedler S, Glasser S, Azani L, Freedman LS, Raziel A, Strassburger D, et al. The effect of medical clowning on pregnancy rates after in vitro fertilization and embryo transfer. *Fertil Steril* 2011; 95(6): 2127-2130.

Chapter 16: Pillar 4 – Toxic substances

1. Organization WH. Tobacco [Internet]. 2022 [cited 2022 Jul 27].
   Available from: www.who.int/news-room/fact-sheets/detail/tobacco
2. Lucas RM, Rodney Harris RM. On the nature of evidence and 'proving' causality: Smoking and lung cancer vs. sun exposure, vitamin D and multiple sclerosis. *Int J Environ Res Public Health* 2018; 15(8): 1726.
   DOI: 10.3390/ijerph15081726
3. Ramlau-Hansen CH, Thulstrup AM, Aggerholm AS, Jensen MC, Toft GBJ. Is smoking a risk factor for decreased semen quality? A cross-sectional analysis. Hum Reprod 2007; 22(1): 188–196.
4. Boeri L, Capogrosso P, Ventimiglia E, Pederzoli F, Cazzaniga W, Chierigo F, et al. Heavy cigarette smoking and alcohol consumption are associated with impaired sperm parameters in primary infertile men. *Asian J Androl* 2019; 21(5): 478-485. DOI: 10.4103/aja.aja_110_18
5. Sansone A, Di Dato C, de Angelis C, Menafra D, Pozza C, Pivonello R, et al. Smoke, alcohol and drug addiction and male fertility. Reproductive Biology and Endocrinology 2018; 16: 3.
   DOI: 10.1186/s12958-018-0320-7
6. De Angelis C, Nardone A, Garifalos F, Pivonello C, Sansone A, Conforti A, et al. Smoke, alcohol and drug addiction and female fertility. *Reproductive Biology and Endocrinology* 2020; 18: 21.
   DOI: 10.1186/s21958-020-0567-7
7. Klzllay DÖ, Aydln C, Aygün AP, Tuhan HÜ, Olukman Ö. Prenatal smoke exposure is associated with increased anogenital distance in female infants: A prospective case-control study. *J Pediatr Endocrinol Metab*

2021; 34(1): 79-88. DOI: 10.1515/jpem-2020-0363

8. [vaping reference - correct?] Szumilas K, Szumilas P, Grzywacz A, Wilk A. The effects of e-cigarette vapor components on the morphology and function of the male and female reproductive systems: A systematic review. *International Journal of Environmental Research and Public Health* 2020: 17(17): 6152. doi: 10.3390/ijerph17176152

9. Sansone A, Di Dato C, de Angelis C, Menafra D, Pozza C, Pivonello R, et al. Smoke, alcohol and drug addiction and male fertility. *Reproductive Biology and Endocrinology* 2018; 15: 3. https://doi.org/10.1186/s12958-018-0320-7

10. De Angelis C, Nardone A, Garifalos F, Pivonello C, Sansone A, Conforti A, et al. Smoke, alcohol and drug addiction and female fertility. *Reproductive Biology and Endocrinology* 2020; 18(1): 21. DOI: 10.1186/s12958-020-0567-7

11. Gunstone B, Piggott L, Butler B, et al. Drinking behaviour and moderation among UK adults: Findings from Drinkaware Monitor 2018 [Internet]. YouGov 2018 p. 1–86. Available from: https://media.drinkaware.co.uk/media/13pb52ms/drinkaware-monitor-2018-report_v100.pdf?v=0.0.9 [cited 2022 Nov 6]

12. Sharma R, Biedenharn KR, Fedor JM, Agarwal A. Lifestyle factors and reproductive health: Taking control of your fertility. *Reproductive Biology and Endocrinology* 2013; 11: 66. DOI: 10.1186/1477-7827-11-66

13. Lyngsø J, Ramlau-Hansen CH, Bay B, Ingerslev HJ, Strandberg-Larsen K, Kesmodel US. Low-to-moderate alcohol consumption and success in fertility treatment: A Danish cohort study. *Hum Reprod* 2019; 34(7): 1334-1344. DOI: 10.1093/humrep/dez050

14. Gormack AA, Peek JC, Derraik JGB, Gluckman PD, Young NL, Cutfield WS. Many women undergoing fertility treatment make poor lifestyle choices that may affect treatment outcome. *Hum Reprod* 2015; 30(7): 1617-1624. DOI: 10.1093/humrep/dev094

15. Setti AS, Halpern G, Braga DP de AF, Iaconelli A, Borges E. Maternal lifestyle and nutritional habits are associated with oocyte quality and ICSI clinical outcomes. *Reprod Biomed Online* 2022; 44(2): 370-379. DOI: 10.1016/j.rbmo.2021.08.025

16. Bai S, Wan Y, Zong L, Li W, Xu X, Zhao Y, et al. Association of Alcohol Intake and Semen Parameters in Men With Primary and Secondary Infertility: A Cross-Sectional Study. *Front Physiol* 2020; 11: Article 56625. DOI: 103389/fphys.2020.566625

17. Lyngsø J, Ramlau-Hansen CH, Bay B, Ingerslev HJ, Hulman A, Kesmodel US. Association between coffee or caffeine consumption and fecundity and fertility: A systematic review and dose-response

meta-analysis. *Clinical Epidemiology* 2017; 9: 699-719.
DOI: 10.2147/CLEP.S146496

18. Mahalingaiah S, Hart JE, Missmer SA. Adult air pollution exposure and risk of infertility in the Nurses Health Study II. *Human Reproduction* 2016; 31(3):;638-647. DOI: 10.1093/humrep/dev330

19. Conforti A, Mascia M, Cioffi G, De Angelis C, Coppola G, De Rosa P, et al. Air pollution and female fertility: A systematic review of literature. *Reproductive Biology and Endocrinology* 2018; 16: 117.
DOI: 10.1186/s12958-018-0433-z

20. Hudda, N. Fruin S. Models for predicting the ratio of particulate pollutant concentrations inside vehicles to roadways. *Environ Sci Technol* 2013; 47(19): 11048–11055.

21. Castellini C, Totaro M, Parisi A, D'Andrea S, Lucente L, Cordeschi G, et al. Bisphenol A and Male Fertility: Myths and Realities. *Frontiers in Endocrinology* 2020; 11: Article 353. DOI: 10.3389/fendo.2020.00353

22. Ragusa A, Svelato A, Santacroce C, Catalano P, Notarstefano V, Carnevali O, et al. Plasticenta: First evidence of microplastics in human placenta. *Environment International* 2021; 146: 106274.
DOI: 10.1016/j.envint.2020.106274

23. Matuszczak E, Komarowska MD, Debek W, Hermanowicz A. The Impact of Bisphenol A on Fertility, Reproductive System, and Development: A Review of the Literature. *International Journal of Endocrinology* 2019; 2019: Article 4068717. DOI: 10.1155/2019/4068717

24. Benson TE, Gaml-Sørensen A, Ernst A, Brix N, Hougaard KS, Hærvig KK, et al. Urinary bisphenol a, f and s levels and semen quality in young adult danish men. *Int J Environ Res Public Health* 2021; 18(4): 1742. DOI: 10.3390/ijerph18041742

25. Kandaraki E, Chatzigeorgiou A, Livadas S, Palioura E, Economou F, Koutsilieris M, et al. Endocrine disruptors and Polycystic Ovary Syndrome (PCOS): Elevated serum levels of bisphenol A in women with PCOS. *J Clin Endocrinol Metab* 2011; 96(3): E480-E484.
DOI: 10.1210/jc2010-1658

26. Chavarro JE, Mínguez-Alarcón L, Chiu YH, Gaskins AJ, Souter I, Williams PL, et al. Soy intake modifies the relation between urinary bisphenol a concentrations and pregnancy outcomes among women undergoing assisted reproduction. *J Clin Endocrinol Metab* 2016; 101(3): 1082-1090. DOI: 10.1210/jc.2015-3473

27. D'Angelo S, Meccariello R. Microplastics: A threat for male fertility. *International Journal of Environmental Research and Public Health* 2021; 18: 2392. DOI 10.3390/ijerph18052392

Chapter 17: Pillar 5 – Sleep

1. UK MH. Sleep and Mental Health [Internet]. [cited 2022 Jul 27]. Available from: https://mentalhealth-uk.org/help-and-information/sleep/#
2. Lateef OM, Akintubosun MO. Sleep and reproductive health. *Journal of Circadian Rhythms* 2020; 18 (1): 1-11. DOI: 10.5334/jcr.190
3. Goldstein CA, Smith YR. Sleep, Circadian Rhythms, and Fertility. *Current Sleep Medicine Reports* 2016; 2: 206-217. DOI: 10.1007/s40675-016-0057-9
4. Gaskin. A, Rich-Edwards. J LC et al. Work schedule and physical factors in relation to fecundity in nurses. *Occup Environ Med* 2015; 72(11): 777–783.
5. Salas-Huetos A, Rosique-Esteban N, Becerra-Tomás N, Vizmanos B, Bulló M, Salas-Salvadó J. The effect of nutrients and dietary supplements on sperm quality parameters: A systematic review andmeta-analysis of randomized clinical trials. *Advances in Nutrition* 2018; 9: 833-848. DOI: 10.1093/ADVANCES/NMY057

Chapter 19: Common fertility nutrition myths

1. Pavan R, Jain S, Shraddha, Kumar A. Properties and Therapeutic Application of Bromelain: A Review. *Biotechnol Res Int* 2012; 2012: Article 976203. DOI: 10.1155/2012/976203
2. Rathnavelu V, Alitheen NB, Sohila S, Kanagesan S, Ramesh R. Potential role of bromelain in clinical and therapeutic applications (Review). *Biomedical Reports* 2016; 5: 283-288. DOI: 10.3892/br.2016.720
3. [clean label project] Protein powder: our point of view [Internet]. Clean Label Project. 2020 Available from: https://cleanlabelproject.org/protein-powder-white-paper/ [cited 2022 Nov 6].

Chapter 20: What supplements should I be taking?

1. Ben-Meir A, Burstein E, Borrego-Alvarez A, Chong J, Wong E, Yavorska T, et al. Coenzyme Q10 restores oocyte mitochondrial function and fertility during reproductive aging. *Aging Cell* 2015; 14(5): 887-895. DOI: 10.1111/acel.12368
2. Florou P, Anagnostis P, Theocharis P, Chourdakis M, Goulis DG. Does coenzyme Q10 supplementation improve fertility outcomes in women

undergoing assisted reproductive technology procedures? A systematic review and meta-analysis of randomized-controlled trials. *Journal of Assisted Reproduction and Genetics* 2020; 37: 2377-2387. DOI: 10.1007/s10815-020-01906-3

3. Schwarze JE, Canales J, Crosby J, Ortega-Hrepich C, Villa S, Pommer R. DHEA use to improve likelihood of IVF/ICSI success in patients with diminished ovarian reserve: A systematic review and meta-analysis. *Jornal Brasileiro de Reproducao Assistida* 2018; 22: 369-374. DOI: 10.5935/1518-0557.20180046

4. Costa M, Canale D, Filicori M, D'lddio S, Lenzi A. L- carnitine in idiopathic asthenozoospermia: a multicenter study. *Andrologia* 1994; 26(3): 155-159. DOI: 10.1111/j.1439-0272.1994.tb00780.x

5. Sigman M, Glass S, Campagnone J, Pryor JL. Carnitine for the treatment of idiopathic asthenospermia: a randomized, double-blind, placebo-controlled trial. *Fertil Steril* 2006; 85(5): 1409-1414. DOI: 10.1016/j.fertnstert.2005.10.055

Further resources

If you would like to read more about the benefits of plant-based nutrition on general health and access easy-to-follow recipes and fact sheets I would recommend the following:

Eating Plant-Based by Dr Shireen Kassam and Dr Zahra Kassam (published by Hammersmith Health Books, 2022)

The Plant Power Doctor by Dr Gemma Newman (her pancakes are a staple in my house!) (published by Ebury Press, 2021)

Plant-Based Nutrition in Clinical Practice edited by Dr Shireen Kassam, Dr Zahra Kassam and Lisa Simon RD (published by Hammersmith Health Books, 2022)

Living PCOS Free by Dr Nitu Bajekal and Rohini Bajekal (published by Hammersmith Health Books, 2022)

Plant Based Health Professionals UK
www.plantbasedhealthprofessionals.com for a wide selection of fantastic fact sheets on key health issues, including fertility, pregnancy and PCOS

Glossary

Adrenaline: The stress hormone that triggers the fight-or-flight response.

AGEs (advanced glycation end products): These harmful compounds are formed when protein or fat combine with sugar in the bloodstream. This process is called glycation.

ALA (alpha-linolenic acid): An essential omega-3 fatty acid found in foods such as walnuts, chia, hemp and flax seeds. Known as the 'parent' omega-3 as it can be converted by the body into the longer chain omega-3 fatty acids EPA and DHA.

Amenorrhoea: Absence of menstrual periods in women of reproductive age.

AMH: A measure of ovarian reserve.

Androgens: Any hormone made by the body that causes characteristics such as excess body hair growth. Testosterone is one of the androgens.

Antioxidants: Any substance that inhibits oxidation – for example, vitamins C and E that neutralise potentially damaging oxidising agents in a living organism.

Antral follicle count: An ultrasound examination taken as part of fertility treatment to evaluate ovarian reserves. When there are fewer antral follicles (small follicles) developing on the ovaries, ovarian reserves are likely to be low, which means fewer eggs.

Asthenozoospermia: The medical term for reduced sperm motility.

Azoospermia: The medical term for the absence of sperm in a man's ejaculate.

Beta-cryptoxanthin: A natural carotenoid and antioxidant found in fruit; it is a precursor of vitamin A in the diet.

Blastocyst: A ball of cells made by the egg around four to five days after it has been fertilised by the sperm; this is the early stage of embryo development.

Beta-carotene: A natural carotenoid and antioxidant found in many fruit and vegetables; it is a precursor of vitamin A in the diet.

Bisphenol A (BPA): An industrial chemical that has been used to make certain plastics and resins since the 1950s.

Body mass index (BMI): A measure based on a person's weight and height to estimate if a person is underweight, at a healthy weight, overweight, or obese. A BMI of 18.5-24.9 is considered a healthy weight, 25-29.9 is considered overweight and 30 or higher is considered obese. It is an imperfect measure but health providers look to the BMI as an added way to monitor weight status.

Cardiovascular disease: A general term to describe a disease of the heart or blood vessels.

Carotenoids: Natural pigments in plants that produce the red, yellow and orange colours in fruit and vegetables and act as antioxidants.

Co-enzyme Q10 (CoQ10): An antioxidant produced by the body and used by its cells for growth and maintenance. It plays an important part in male and female fertility.

Cortisol: An important hormone with several roles, including regulating the body's stress response.

DHA (docosahexaenoic acid): An omega-3 fatty acid important for sperm quality and improved fertility treatment outcomes.

DHEA (dehydroepiandrosterone): A steroid hormone produced naturally in the body that can be used to make other hormones, including testosterone and oestrogen. It is involved in ovarian follicle development and oocyte quality.

D-chiro-inositol (DCI): A molecule used in clinical practice to induce ovulation in women with PCOS.

Endocrine system: The body's hormone system which controls or regulates many biological processes.

Endometriosis: A chronic condition where tissue similar to the lining of the womb grows in other places, such as the ovaries and fallopian tubes.

Endorphins: Neurotransmitters released by the brain to alleviate pain and promote feelings of pleasure.

EPA (eicosapentaenoic acid): An omega-3 fatty acid important for sperm quality and improved fertility treatment outcomes.

Epididymis: A tube attached to the testes where the sperm are stored.

Erectile dysfunction: The inability to achieve and maintain an erection.

Ethnicity: Belonging to a population group or subgroup made up of people who share a common cultural background or descent.

Fallopian tubes: The pair of tubes along which eggs travel from the ovaries to the uterus. Fertilisation takes place in either one of the Fallopian tubes but the zygote produced must travel back to the uterus to implant and grow. If this happens mistakenly in a

Fallopian tube, what is called an ectopic pregnancy occurs which has no hope of going to term and is very dangerous to the mother if not stopped naturally or by surgical intervention.

Folate/folic acid: A water-soluble B-vitamin (vitamin B9) that plays an essential role in fertility and early pregnancy and is found in large amounts in green leafy vegetables.

Free radical(s): Highly reactive and unstable molecules made by the body naturally as a by-product of normal metabolism and which need to be balanced out be antioxidants.

FSH (follicle stimulating hormone): A hormone made by the pituitary gland in the brain that stimulates the follicles in the ovaries from which eggs are released, thereby helping an egg to mature.

Functional hypothalamic amenorrhoea (FHA): A functional disorder of the hypothalamus in the brain which has an impact on the hormones it produces resulting in the absence of menstruation.

GnRH (gonadotrophin releasing hormone): The hormone responsible for the release of FSH and LH from the pituitary gland in the brain.

Healthful plant-based diet index (hPDI): A plant-based scoring system that gives positive points for healthy plant-based foods and negative points to animal foods and less healthful plant-based foods such as sugar sweetened beverages and refined grains.

Haem iron: The type of iron found in animal foods which is associated with an increased risk of ovulatory infertility.

Hyperandrogenism: A medical condition characterised by high circulating levels of androgens, including testosterone, in women resulting in symptoms such as head hair loss and increase in body hair.

Hyperinsulinaemia: High levels of insulin in the body that can affect blood glucose levels and is strongly associated with the development of type 2 diabetes.

Hypothalamus: A small region of the brain located at the base of the brain. It has many important roles including releasing GnRH, a hormone that enables the pituitary gland to release important reproductive hormones such as LH and FSH.

Implantation: The process whereby a fertilised egg(s) burrows into the uterus lining.

Infertility: The inability to get pregnant after 12 months or more of regular unprotected sexual intercourse.

Inositol: A kind of sugar the body makes, found in foods such as fruit (especially citrus fruit), beans, whole grains and nuts. Inositol is also available in supplement form and is used as a treatment for PCOS where insulin resistance is present. Also known as myo-inositol (MI).

Insulin resistance: When cells in the body are unable to respond to insulin and therefore cannot take up glucose. This is the main cause of type 2 diabetes but occurs in a number of related conditions, including PCOS.

Intracytoplasmic sperm injection (ICSI): A form of fertility treatment where the highest quality sperm are directly injected into the uterus where they are left to fertilise the eggs naturally.

In vitro fertilisation (IVF): A form of fertility treatment where sperm are introduced to an egg in a laboratory to fertilise it and the fertilised egg is then returned to the woman's womb as an embryo.

Leaky gut: Excess gut wall permeability allowing larger molecules to enter the bloodstream than would be allowed by a healthy gut lining.

Leydig cells: Specialised cells in the testicles which produce testosterone.

LGBTQIA+: An inclusive term that encompasses people of all genders and sexualities: lesbian, gay, bisexual, transgender, queer, intersex, asexual plus members of other supportive communities.

LH (luteinising hormone): A hormone essential for healthy reproduction in both men and women. In women LH works with FSH to enable a healthy menstrual cycle and trigger ovulation. In men it triggers testosterone production.

Lignans: Fibre-associated compounds found in plant foods, with high concentrations found in flaxseeds.

Lutein: A carotenoid with a deep yellow pigment.

Macronutrients: The types of food (carbohydrates, proteins and fats) needed in large amounts in the diet.

Meta-analysis: The examination of data from a number of independent studies of the same subject, in order to determine overall trends.

Methylenetetrahydrofolate reductase: A key enzyme of folate (vitamin B9) metabolism.

Microbiome: The collective term for the genetic makeup of the micro-organisms known as microbiota.

Microbiota: A collection of micro-organisms, including fungi, bacteria and viruses, that are most concentrated in the large intestine (colon).

Micronutrients: Vitamins and minerals needed in small quantities for normal growth and development.

Monounsaturated fatty acids (MUFAs): A type of unsaturated fat, important for female fertility found, for example, in olive oil and avocados.

MTHFR: An enzyme that breaks down the amino acid homocysteine. A genetic abnormality can result in high levels of homocysteine and low folate levels which can negatively impact fertility and pregnancy outcomes.

Oestradiol: A major oestrogen produced in the ovaries.

Oestrogen: One of the main female sex hormones, although men also produce it in smaller amounts. There are three different oestrogens: oestradiol, oestrone and oestriol.

Oligospermia: The medical term for a low sperm concentration.

Oligoasthenospermia: The medical term for low sperm concentration and poor motility.

Oligozoospermia: The medical term for a low sperm count where the man has less than 15 million sperm per millilitre of semen.

Omega-3 fatty acids: A blanket term for ALA (alpha-linolenic acid – the type found in plant foods), EPA and DHA (the types found in fish and algae supplements). They are essential fatty acids as they are not produced naturally within the human body and a good dietary intake is needed. Omega-3 fatty acids are important, among many other things, for brain health, the normal functioning of organs and for sperm quality.

Omega-6 fatty acids: These are another type of essential fatty acid that occur naturally in many plant foods, such as vegetables, nuts and vegetable oils. As omega-6 and omega-3 compete for absorption, it is important not to over-consume omega-6 at the expense of omega-3. The ideal balance is thought to be 4:1 of omega-6 to omega-3. [OK?]

Ovaries: The paired female glands in which the eggs are formed, ready to be released during ovulation, and where the hormones oestrogen and progesterone are made.

Oxalates: Naturally occurring compounds in some plant foods that can reduce absorption of minerals, including calcium and iron.

Oxidative stress: An imbalance between free radicals and antioxidants in the body which can lead to cell and DNA damage, including the DNA in the sperm and egg.

PCOS (polycystic ovary syndrome or PCOD): Terms used interchangeably for an endocrine (hormone) disorder affecting ovarian function that is strongly associated with insulin resistance.

Phytates: Antioxidant compounds found in some plant foods that can bind with certain minerals, including zinc, iron and calcium, to slow their absorption.

Phytonutrients (or phytochemicals): The compounds in or derived from plants that have health benefits both to the plant itself and to humans.

Phyto-oestrogens: Plant oestrogens, including isoflavones and lignans. They are found in several different types of food, including soya, grains, beans and some fruit and vegetables.

Polyphenols: Compounds naturally found in plants that have antioxidant and anti-inflammatory properties and are associated with the colours of fruit and vegetables; they include the carotenoids.

Polyunsaturated fats: A type of unsaturated fat with multiple double-bonds in their chemical make-up; these include omega-3 and omega-6 fatty acids.

Progesterone: A type of steroid hormone that plays an important part in the menstrual cycle and early stages of pregnancy.

Race v. ethnicity: Race is usually associated with biology and linked with physical characteristics such as hair and skin colour. Ethnicity is linked with cultural expression and identification.

Randomised control study/trial: A research study that measures the effectiveness of an intervention or treatment. The participants are randomly assigned to either the intervention arm or placebo arm which is the control group.

Reproductive age: From the start of a woman's first period until menopause is reached aged around 51.

Rotterdam criteria: A tool used to clinically diagnose PCOS.

Saturated fats: Dietary fats that are generally solid at room temperature and contain no double-bonds in their chemical make-up. They are negatively associated with health and fertility outcomes.

Semen/seminal fluid: A mix of sperm and fluids produced in the seminiferous tubules of the testes.

Seminiferous tubules: Small coiled tubes inside the testes responsible for producing sperm.

Sertoli cells: Cells in the seminiferous tubules of the testes essential for sperm production.

Sex hormone binding globulin (SHBH): A protein produced by the liver that attaches itself to sex hormones, including testosterone, controlling how much of these hormones is delivered to the body's tissues. A blood SHBG test tells us if there is too much or too little testosterone available for use by the body.

Scrotum: The bag of skin that holds and helps to protect the testicles. It acts as a temperature controller for the testicles which need to be about 2<degrees>C less than normal body temperature. In order to facilitate this the scrotum will contract or relax its muscles to bring the testicles closer to the body for warmth or further away to allow them to cool.

Short chain fatty acids (SCFAs): Fatty acids are the building blocks of fats/oils and come in different lengths. SCFAs are produced when the friendly bacteria in the gut ferment fibre in the colon.

Sperm: A single sperm is the male reproductive cell that consists of three main parts: the head, mid-section and tail. When a sperm penetrates an egg fertilisation occurs.

Subfertility: The inability to get pregnant within 12 months of trying to conceive.

Systematic review: A type of review of existing research to examine the quality of the evidence presented to enable the researchers to answer their question making use of all available data.

Teratospermia: The medical term for a low percentage of normal sperm.

Testicles/testes: The pair of organs found inside the scrotum, responsible for making testosterone and generating sperm.

Testosterone: A type of androgen, produced in larger quantities in males but also produced by females and in larger amounts in PCOS and is responsible for PCOS symptoms such as excess body and facial hair, acne and head-hair thinning/loss.

Trans fats: A type of unsaturated fat produced in both natural and artificial forms, associated with adverse health and fertility outcomes.

Uterus: Traditionally known as the womb, the hollow organ inside a woman's pelvis where a fertilised egg implants and the foetus grows and develops.

Unsaturated fats: These include monounsaturated and polyunsaturated fats and are associated with improved male and female fertility outcomes. In men, polyunsaturated fatty acids are associated with improved sperm quality and in women monounsaturated fatty acids are associated with higher fertility rates and a reduced chance of pre-term delivery, and play a role in foetal development.

Vagina: The tube-like structure surrounded by muscles that leads from the uterus to the outside of the body.

Vas deferens/sperm duct: The tube which carries sperm from the epididymis to the penis.

Vulva: The external female genital area.

WFBP (whole food plant-based): A term to describe a dietary pattern that excludes animal products and focuses on eating plant-based foods in their whole form rather than processed varieties.

WHO (World Health Organization): A part of the United Nations that deals with major health issues around the world.

Zeaxanthin: A deep yellow carotenoid pigment found in plants.

Index

*Page numbers in bold refer to entries in the Glossary.

Index

*Page numbers in bold refer to entries in the Glossary.

*Page numbers in bold refer to entries in the Glossary.

*Page numbers in bold refer to entries in the Glossary.

Index

Index

*Page numbers in bold refer to entries in the Glossary.

Index

*Page numbers in bold refer to entries in the Glossary.

Index

*Page numbers in bold refer to entries in the Glossary.

Patient testimonials

'We had been trying to conceive for five years. I did fall pregnant eventually but sadly miscarried. I was willing to try anything to boost our chances as we were about to start IVF.

'I thought I was really healthy: I'm a nurse and a yoga teacher and I have a degree in nutrition. I thought there probably wasn't anything I didn't already know but I wanted to cover all bases.

'Under Lisa's care I feel healthier than I ever have. I have so much more energy and my hormonal acne and headaches have disappeared. I'm convinced that Lisa's dietary advice helped me throughout the grueling IVF process as I felt balanced and well. Our first round of IVF worked and we now have a beautiful baby girl!

'Working with Lisa was such a positive experience. She was so professional and knowledgeable and helped me cut through all the dubious and outdated dietary information there is out there.

'I feel so grateful I came across Lisa and a fully plant-based diet and definitely feel this had a huge impact on the outcome for us.'

Gemma

'My husband and I have worked with a range of different dietitians, nutritional therapists, doctors and other health professionals. Lisa has been the one who has really stood out from the rest. She has been the only one to make us feel truly calm and reassured, which has been the greatest gift. During a very stressful time she has given us really sound advice which is evidence-based and helped us feel as though we could trust our diets as well as our bodies again. She has given us really practical and clear advice on how to meet all our nutritional needs. I cannot adequately express how invaluable her support has been to us. Working with her has freed us from a great deal of stress and we feel so much more positive and hopeful as we prepare for fertility treatment.'

Cait

'My consultation with Lisa has helped enormously. Initially I had some concerns with following a plant-based diet in pregnancy, but she has reassured me so much and given me such helpful advice. I am now confident in what I am eating and how to optimise my nutrition during this stage. Lisa was so lovely, friendly and encouraging, I would absolutely recommend her to anyone looking for advice and help with their diet'

Gemma S

Also from Hammersmith Health Books...

Living PCOS Free

How to regain your hormonal health and go from surviving to thriving with Polycystic Ovary Syndrome

By Dr Nitu Bajekal and Rohini Bajekal

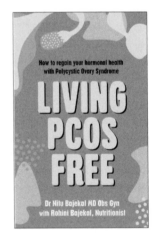

This practical guide will show you how to identify and successfully manage this common but under-diagnosed condition using proven lifestyle approaches alongside western medicine. With over 35 years of clinical experience, Dr Nitu Bajekal, AKA 'the 'Plant-Based Gynae,' and Nutritionist Rohini Bajekal, break through misinformation, providing clarity and support to help you tackle your symptoms - from irregular periods to acne and anxiety.

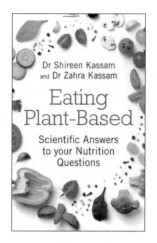

Also from Hammersmith Health Books...

Plant-Based Nutrition in Clinical Practice

Edited by Dr Shireen Kassam, Dr Zahra Kassam
and Lisa Simon RD

with a team of 27 contributing specialist authors

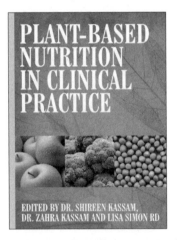

In *Plant-Based Nutrition in Clinical Practice*, a team of specialist
authors, edited by two hospital doctors and registered dietitian
Lisa Simon, curate the current knowledge base that supports
a whole food, plant-based diet as the best way to address both
individual and planetary health. Taking both a holistic and
systems-based approach, the book presents the uses, benefits
and practical application of a plant-based diet to support
patient care, disease prevention and management.